Pulmonary Management
in Physical Therapy

CLINICS IN PHYSICAL THERAPY

EDITORIAL BOARD

Otto D. Payton, Ph.D., **Chairman**
Louis R. Amundsen, Ph.D.
Suzann K. Campbell, Ph.D.

Forthcoming Volumes in the Series

**Physical Therapy Assessment in
Early Infancy**
Irma J. Wilhelm, M.S., P.T., guest editor

Physical Therapy of the Low Back, 2nd Ed.
Lance T. Twomey, Ph.D., and James R. Taylor, M.D.,
Ph. D., guest editors

Pulmonary Management in Physical Therapy

Edited by
Cynthia Coffin Zadai, M.S., P.T.

Assistant Professor
Program in Physical Therapy
Massachusetts General Hospital Institute
 of Health Professions
Director
Rehabilitation Services
Beth Israel Hospital
Boston, Massachusetts

CHURCHILL LIVINGSTONE
New York, Edinburgh, London, Melbourne, Tokyo

WF
145
P98145
1992

Library of Congress Cataloging-in-Publication Data

Pulmonary management in physical therapy / edited by Cynthia Coffin Zadai.
     p.   cm.—(Clinics in physical therapy)
   Includes bibliographical references and index.
   ISBN: 0-443-08741-5
   1. Lungs—Diseases—Physical therapy. 2. Respiratory therapy.
I. Zadai, Cynthia Coffin. II. Series.
   [DNLM: 1. Cardiovascular Diseases—therapy. 2. Lung—
physiopathology. 3. Lung Diseases—therapy. 4. Physical Therapy—
methods. 5. Respiratory Function Tests. WF 145 P98145]
   RC735.P58P85 1992
   615.8'2—dc20
   DNLM/DLC
   for Library of Congress   92-49637
                                                CIP

© **Churchill Livingstone Inc. 1992**

Distributed in the United Kingdom by Churchill Livingstone, Robert Stevenson House, 1–3 Baxter's Place, Leith Walk, Edinburgh EH1 3AF, and by associated companies, branches, and representatives throughout the world.

Accurate indications, adverse reactions, and dosage schedules for drugs are provided in this book, but it is possible that they may change. The reader is urged to review the package information data of the manufacturers of the medications mentioned.

The Publishers have made every effort to trace the copyright holders for borrowed material. If they have inadvertently overlooked any, they will be pleased to make the necessary arrangements at the first opportunity.

Acquisitions Editor: *Leslie Burgess*
Copy Editor: *Katharine Leawanna O'Moore*
Production Designer: *Jody L. Ouellette*
Production Supervisor: *Jeanine Furino*

Printed in the United States of America

First published in 1992   7 6 5 4 3 2 1

Contributors

Linda D. Crane, M.M.Sc., P.T., C.C.S.
Instructor, Division of Physical Therapy, Department of Orthopaedics and Rehabilitation, University of Miami School of Medicine, Miami, Florida

Elizabeth Dean, Ph.D., P.T.
Assistant Professor, School of Rehabilitation Medicine, University of British Columbia Faculty of Medicine, Vancouver, British Columbia, Canada

Scot Irwin, M.S., P.T., C.C.S.
Instructor, Division of Rehabilitation Medicine, Department of Physical Therapy, Emory University School of Medicine, Atlanta, Georgia; Director, Rehabilitation Services, Southern Regional Medical Center, Riverdale, Georgia

Claudia R. Levenson, M.S., P.T.
Clinical Director, Department of Chest Physical Therapy, Beth Israel Hospital, Boston, Massachusetts

Denise F. Patrick, M.S., P.T.
Former Director, Outpatient Chest Clinic, Beth Israel Hospital, Boston, Massachusetts

Jocelyn Ross, B.S.R., M.Sc., P.T.
Research Associate, School of Rehabilitation Medicine, University of British Columbia Faculty of Medicine; Physiotherapist, Rehabilitation Services, Vancouver General Hospital, Vancouver, British Columbia, Canada

Julie A. Starr, M.S., P.T.
Clinical Assistant Professor, Department of Physical Therapy, Sargent College of Allied Health Professions, Boston University, Boston, Massachusetts

Cynthia Coffin Zadai, M.S., P.T.
Assistant Professor, Program in Physical Therapy, Massachusetts General Hospital Institute of Health Professions; Director, Rehabilitation Services, Beth Israel Hospital, Boston, Massachusetts

Preface

Physical therapy (PT) management of patients with pulmonary impairment has traditionally been considered a "specialty" component of PT practice in the United States, one most commonly performed by a separate group of physical therapists labeled "chest PTs." In fact, the label *chest PT* has also become a descriptor of a wide variety of treatment techniques predominantly used to achieve airway clearance (e.g., percussion, vibration, and postural drainage), further confounding the issue in pulmonary care of "who is doing what to whom and what is the goal?"

The separation of pulmonary PT from general PT practice has furthered the misconception that evaluation of the pulmonary system is not an integral portion of every PT examination. Similarly, the treatment techniques are also considered different and separate, when in many instances they are the same techniques as those used to treat musculoskeletal dysfunction resulting from neurologic, orthopedic, and cardiac impairment. *Pulmonary Management in Physical Therapy* seeks to emphasize that pulmonary assessment is an integral portion of the PT examination performed by either the generalist or specialty PT practitioner. Pulmonary impairment may in fact be identified as "musculoskeletal" in ventilatory pump abnormality, "pathophysiologic" in gas exchange abnormality, or "functional" in reduced oxygen uptake during activities of daily living. Hence, PT management may include positioning to decrease the musculoskeletal work of breathing, breathing exercises to improve ventilation/perfusion ratios, or cycle ergometry to increase oxygen uptake and cardiovascular endurance.

Consequently, this text presents the pulmonary system information in a format that promotes use by PT generalists or specialists across a broad spectrum of physical disorders. The initial chapters describe the musculoskeletal ventilatory pump and its relationship to gas exchange both at rest and during activity. The physiologic specifics of normal and abnormal cardiopulmonary response to increased oxygen demand in any subject are described in Chapters 2 and 3. This information provides the background data to evaluate and measure adequacy of cardiopulmonary function as described in Chapter 4.

Chapters 5 through 8 review the wide variety of therapeutic interventions currently available to treat cardiopulmonary system impairment. The chapters group treatment techniques as they are typically used in combination to achieve a common goal or as they are commonly reviewed in the literature. Each technique is defined and described prior to discussion of clinical indicators, considerations for use, and what is known or not known regarding technique efficacy in specific patient populations.

Chapter 9 summarizes the material presented by reviewing the clinical decision making process and applying it to evaluation and treatment of pulmonary impairment. Three cases are included that represent multisystem impairment and the need to integrate evaluation and treatment of pulmonary impairment into routine PT evaluation and treatment.

This book is intended as a reference for the practicing clinician. Terminology is defined whenever possible to clarify the context of use for evaluation and treatment techniques. An attempt has been made to separate the clinical practice from the clinician and to integrate pulmonary care into the broader scope of general PT practice.

Cynthia Coffin Zadai, M.S., P.T.

Acknowledgments

I would like to acknowledge and thank:

Colleen Kigin, Scot Irwin, Ray Blessey, Shirley Sahrmann, Steve Rose, Alan Jette, Pam Catlin, Helen Hislop, and Sandy Burkhart, who helped me to see physical therapy in my patient care.

The authors, who worked long and hard to put this book together in the most relevant way to meet the needs of the practicing physical therapist . . . while they continued to practice.

The infinite patience and support of my co-workers at Beth Israel.

Leslie Burgess at Churchill Livingstone, who was positive, supportive, and waited, and waited, and waited . . . and still understood.

My family, who is *always* there.

Contents

1 | Functional Anatomy and Physiology of Ventilation

Linda D. Crane

The structure and function of the ventilatory pump is complex and wonderfully efficient in carrying out its multitude of functions. The primary function is breathing, or ventilation ($\dot{V}e$), which provides a mechanism for introducing O_2 and expelling CO_2. The importance of $\dot{V}e$ can not be overemphasized, as it is the first essential component of the total gas delivery system on which the body depends to function both at rest and during exercise.[1] Other functions that depend on proper function of the ventilatory pump include speech, singing, and any other controlled breathing activity. Respiratory or ventilatory muscles also are involved in stabilization of the shoulder girdle; movements of the trunk, neck; and back; maintaining posture; defecation; and parturition.[2]

Many health care professionals, as well as the general public, have incomplete or outdated information about the functions of the ventilatory pump, especially regarding the functions of specific muscles that contribute to $\dot{V}e$. There is also much controversy within the scientific community regarding the actions and roles of some ventilatory muscles. One controversy dates back to the 1700s and involves the intercostal muscles.[3] Sophisticated electromyographic (EMG), radiographic, and motion analysis technologies have not yet solved the difficulties analyzing the specific and integrated components and motions of the ventilatory pump.

This chapter reviews the structure and functions of the normal ventilatory pump, and attempts to combine the old and new information available in the literature. The musculoskeletal anatomy of the ventilatory pump is described, with emphasis on the functional and biomechanical consequences of the structures' composition, orientation, and locations. The actions of the ventilatory

1

muscles are presented according to their activity during quiet versus forced breathing and inspiration versus expiration. The mechanics of breathing are discussed with respect to the integration and coordination of the actions and motions of the chest wall. The end of this chapter presents a discussion of the effects of age, posture, and changes in lung volume and load on chest wall mechanics in normal, healthy individuals; this provides the reader with a source of comparison for later chapters on the effects of exercise, disease, and dysfunction on the lungs and ventilatory pump.

STRUCTURE OF THE VENTILATORY PUMP

The chest wall is generally considered to consist of three parts: the rib cage with its musculature, the diaphragm, and the abdomen with its musculature.[4,5] However, the chest wall is actually an "anatomic and physiologic abstraction" because its functions are determined by all the structures outside the lungs that are active or move during breathing.[6]

Skeletal Framework

The rib cage provides a rigid protection to the thoracic structures and generally comprises the manubriosternum, twelve pairs of ribs, costal cartilages, and twelve thoracic vertebrae and their intervertebral discs. The shape and structure of the rib cage change significantly as the newborn infant matures to adulthood. Infants' ribs are primarily cartilaginous and run horizontally, and their rib cages (horizontal cross section) are circular. The ribs gradually ossify, and the thoracic shape changes from a larger anteroposterior to a larger lateral diameter.[7,8] The change in shape is likely a result of the effects of gravity (especially as the growing child assumes an upright position) and of the actions of the ventilatory muscles on the rib cage.

The 12 thoracic vertebral bodies are wedge-shaped, with their posterior aspects approximately 1 to 2 mm higher than their anterior aspects. This wedging configuration results in the primary kyphotic curve of the thoracic vertebral column. The bony contribution to the primary thoracic kyphosis is furthered by the relatively thin and parallel intervertebral discs and disc spaces (unlike the cervical and lumbar regions, which have large disc–to–vertebral-body–thickness ratios).[9]

The 12 pairs of ribs articulate posteriorly with the bodies and transverse processes of the thoracic vertebrae and their intervertebral discs. The rib heads of ribs 2–10 articulate with two adjacent thoracic vertebrae and the intervertebral disc via an intra-articular ligament at the costovertebral (CV) joints. Ribs 1, 11, and 12 articulate with only one facet on the body of their corresponding thoracic vertebrae, making these costovertebral joints more mobile.[9,10]

The tubercles of ribs 1–10 articulate with facets on the anterior ends of the vertebral spinous processes, forming the costotransverse (CT) joints. For ribs

2–10, the CT articulation is with the lowermost of the two vertebrae to which the rib head is connected contributing to the oblique angulation of the ribs (Fig. 1-1).[11]

Ribs 1–10 attach anteriorly to the costal cartilages at costochondral articulations (Fig. 1-2). Ribs 1–7 are so-called true ribs because their costal cartilages articulate with the manubriosternum. The cartilages of ribs 8–10 articulate with the cartilages immediately above them. Ribs 11 and 12 are "floating" ribs and do not articulate anteriorly.[9–11] The CV, CT, and chondrosternal joints are all synovial joints (with the exception of the first chondrosternal joint, which is a synchondrosis) up to middle age.[11]

The sternum has three sections: the manubrium, the body of the sternum, and the xiphoid process. These sections are joined by synchrondrotic articulations (similar to symphysis pubis), which tend to ossify later in life. The ribs are thin, elastic, and curvilinear. They change in shape and obliquity from superior to inferior due to the differences in shape and to the in situ orientations of the ribs.[9,11]

Ventilatory Muscle Structure

Discussion of the ventilatory muscles in this chapter is organized according to inspiratory and expiratory functions. Some of these muscles are active or inactive at times, depending on level of physical activity, disease state, and the

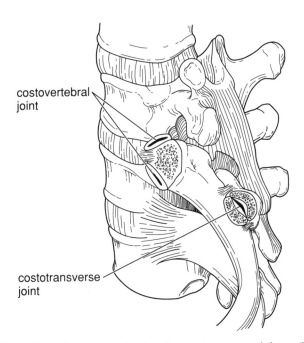

costovertebral joint

costotransverse joint

Fig. 1-1. Relationship of costovertebral and costotransverse joints. (From Fam and Smythe,[10] with permission.)

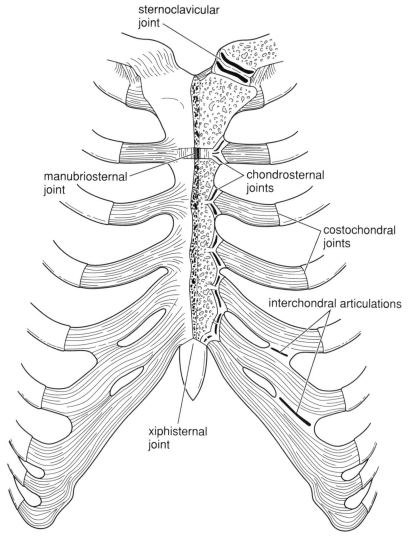

Fig. 1-2.   Skeletal anatomy of the anterior chest wall. (From Fam and Smythe,[10] with permission.)

specific goal of the ventilatory action (e. g., coughing, blowing out candles, maintaining uninterrupted speech). This section briefly reviews ventilatory muscle anatomy.

Muscles of Inspiration

Diaphragm.   The diaphragm is the primary muscle of inspiration for any ventilatory function. The diaphragm is a unique skeletal muscle because the fibers arising from various peripheral circumferential structures insert into a central tendon (Fig. 1-3).[5] The central tendon is a noncontractile tendinous aponeurosis located just below the pericardium, to which it is partly attached. The central tendon is roughly boomerang-shaped and has three parts: the middle, right, and left leaflets.[11,12]

Muscle fibers of the diaphragm radiate and descend from the central tendon and form the *costal* and *crural* parts of the muscle. These portions appear to have different embryologic origins and they definitely have different functions.[2,13] The diaphragm is roughly dome-shaped, with the central tendon as the apex.

The crural, or vertebral portions of the diaphragm insert on the anterolateral bodies of L1–L3 and the aponeurotic medial (psoas) and lateral (quadratus lumborum) arcuate ligaments.[2,8,11] The costal portions insert on the posterior xiphoid process and posterior upper margins of the lower six ribs. The costal fibers are vertically aligned as they continue from their insertions cranially toward the central tendon. The apposed relationship of these fibers and the inner aspect of the lower rib cage is called the zone of apposition (Fig. 1-4).[5,8] Motor innervation of the diaphragm arises from spinal cord levels C3–C5 and

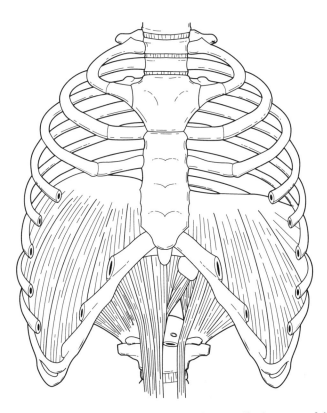

Fig. 1-3. Representation of configuration of the human diaphragm at full expiration. (From Trans. Am. Clin. Climatol. Assoc. 83:200, 1981, with permission.)

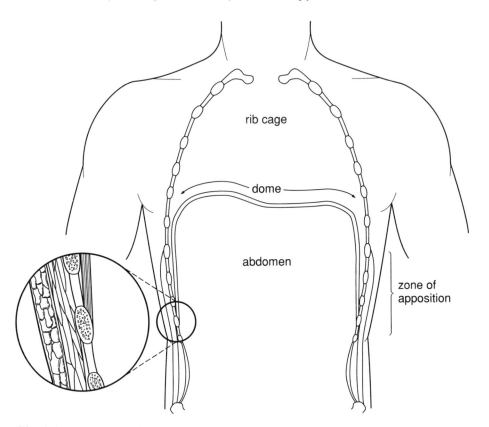

Fig. 1-4.   Frontal section of the chest wall at full expiration. (From De Troyer and Estenne,[5] with permission.)

travels to the right and left hemidiaphragms via the right and left phrenic nerves (no intercostal motor innervation).[5] Blood supply to the diaphragm is from the internal mammary, intercostal, and superior and inferior phrenic arteries.[14]

Muscle fiber type composition has a great influence on fatigue resistance and functional performance of a muscle. The functions or activities of a muscle may influence fiber type composition in turn. The diaphragm is generally accepted to be composed of three types of muscle fibers, at least 75 percent of which are fatigue-resistant. Approximately 55 percent of the fibers in the adult diaphragm are slow twitch oxidative (SO) and highly resistant to fatigue. Twenty to 25 percent of the fibers are fast twitch oxidative, glycolytic (FOG) and although intermediate, are quite fatigue-resistant. The remainder of the muscle is fast twitch glycolytic (FG) and very susceptible to fatigue.[15-17]

Intercostal Muscles.   The structure of the intercostal muscles is well known, but the action of these muscles is very controversial and is discussed in detail later in this chapter. As with many muscles, the anatomic arrangement of the intercostals does not completely reveal their functions but does form a basis for study and theory. The intercostals include the *internal* and *external* intercostals, which are two thin layers of muscle that occupy the intercostal spaces and are named according to their relationship to each other.[11]

The external intercostals extend posteriorly from the tubercles of the ribs to the costochondral junction, where they thin and form the anterior intercostal membrane. The alignment of the external intercostals, when viewed anteriorly, is similar to a V. The internal intercostals extend from the sternocostal junctions anteriorly to the angles of the ribs, where they thin and form the posterior intercostal membrane. The fiber alignment of the internal intercostals, when viewed anteriorly, is similar to an upside-down V. These two muscle layers are roughly perpendicular to each other (Fig. 1-5). The portions of the internal intercostals close to the sternum are the intercartilaginous or parasternals. The remainder of the internal intercostals is referred to as the lateral and posterior, or interosseous, portion.[5,8,11]

The intercostals are innervated by the intercostal nerves, which arise from spinal cord levels T1–T12. Arterial blood supply to the upper two intercostal spaces are by the superior intercostal artery branch of the subclavian. The second space is also supplied by a branch from the first aortic intercostal artery. The intercostal arteries (branches of the aorta) and the anterior intercostal branches of the internal mammary arteries supply the remainder of the intercostal muscles.[8,11] The intercostal muscles also have three fiber types with a percent distribution very similar to the diaphragm. The intercostals are 53 percent SO, 26 percent FOG, and 21 percent FG fibers.[18]

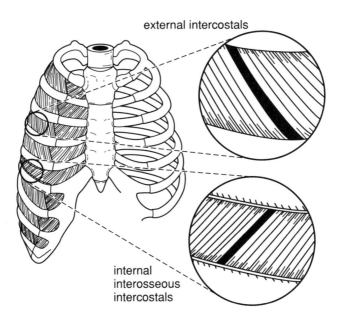

external intercostals

internal interosseous intercostals

Fig. 1-5. Muscle fiber alignments of the external and internal intercostals. (From De Troyer and Estenne,[5] with permission.)

Scalenes. The scalene muscles are primary muscles of inspiration, not just accessory muscles as previously thought.[2,19] The scalenes arise from the anterior tubercles of the transverse processes of C3–C7. The anterior and medius insert on the superior surface of rib 1. The posterior scalene muscle inserts on upper rib 2. The scalenes are innervated by the anterior divisions of the lower cervical nerves arising from C2–C7. Arterial blood supply is via the ascending cervical branch of the inferior thyroid, which is a branch of the subclavian artery.[2,8,11,20] Muscle fiber composition of the scalenes is 60 percent SO, 23 percent FOG, and 17 percent FG.[18]

Sternocleidomastoid. The sternocleidomastoid (SCM) muscles are important accessory muscles of inspiration that have significant ventilatory functions. Each SCM muscle arises by two heads from the clavicle and sternum, which blend with each other, and inserts onto the outer surface of the mastoid process. Innervation of the SCM muscles is by the spinal accessory nerves and the second cervical nerves. Arterial blood supply is from the superior thyroid branch of the external carotid artery.[8,11]

Other Accessory Muscles of Inspiration include the trapezius, pectoralis major, and minor, serratus anterior, latissimus dorsi, and other muscles that insert onto the rib cage and the shoulder girdle. There is little information regarding the activity of these accessory muscles during breathing under different conditions. Many of these muscles appear anatomically to be potential inspiratory muscles, but their individual or combined actions have not been demonstrated except under extreme or unique circumstances presented by exertion, disease, and deformity.[8,21]

Levatores Costarum. The levatores costarum are active during inspiration but likely do not significantly contribute to elevation of the ribs because they form inefficient third-class levers with extremely long resistance arms. The levatores costarum arise from the transverse process of C7–T11 and insert onto the next lowest rib between the tubercle and angle of the rib. These muscles are innervated by the intercostal nerves and receive their blood supply from the posterior intercostal arteries.[8,20]

Muscles of Expiration

Abdominals. The abdominal muscles are accessory muscles of expiration, but they also contribute to inspiration in various ways that will be discussed later. The abdominal muscles include the rectus abdominis, internal and external obliques, and transversus abdominis. The attachments, innervation, and blood supply of these muscles are presented in Table 1-1.

Triangularis Sterni. The triangularis sterni (TS), or sternocostalis or transverse thoracis, is a primary expiratory muscle that contributes to active expiration.[22] The TS is a thin, flat muscle deep to the internal intercostals. It arises from the lower sternum and sternal ends of the lower true rib costal cartilages, and inserts by digitations into the inner surfaces of the costal cartilages of ribs 2–6.[11] Innervation is via the internal intercostal nerves from spinal cord levels T7–L1 and blood supply from the internal thoracic and intercostal arteries.[9,11,20]

Table 1-1. Attachments, Innervation, and Blood Supply of the Abdominal Muscles

Muscle	Superior Attachment	Inferior Attachment	Innervation	Blood Supply
Rectus abdominis	Anterior surface xiphoid process and 5th–7th costal cartilages	Pubic crest and pubic symphysis	Lower 6 intercostal; iliohypogastric; ilioinguinal	Muscular branch of superior and inferior epigastric
External oblique	External surfaces of ribs 5–12	Anterior 1/2 of iliac crest; aponeurosis of anterior abdominal wall	Lower 6 thoracic and upper 2 lumbar	Muscular branch of superior and inferior epigastric
Internal oblique	8th–10th costal cartilages; aponeurosis from 10th costal cartilage to pubis forming linea alba	Lumbar fascia; anterior ⅔ of iliac crest; lateral ⅔ of inguinal ligament	Lower intercostal; iliohypogastric; ilioinguinal	Muscular branches of superior and inferior epigastric; deep circumflex iliac
Transversus abdominis (or transversalis)	Inner surface of 5th–10th costal cartilages; lumbar fascia; anterior ⅔ of iliac crest; lateral ⅓ of inguinal ligament	Aponeurotic sheath into linea alba	Lower 6 intercostal; iliohypogastric; ilioinguinal	Deep circumflex iliac; inferior epigastric

Quadratus Lumborum. Its functions, which will be described later, are very different from those of the other expiratory muscles. The quadratus lumborum arises from the crest of the ileum and iliolumbar ligament and attaches to the inferior margin of rib 12 and the transverse processes of L1–L4. The muscles are innervated by the spinal nerves from approximately T12–L3 and receive their blood supply from the lumbar branch of the iliolumbar artery.[9,11,20,21]

FUNCTIONS OF THE VENTILATORY MUSCLES

Gender Differences

There is no evidence of differing anatomic arrangements or recruitment of the ventilatory muscles between males and females. Although the reader may still occasionally find a reference to differences in ventilatory mechanics between the genders,[26] no differences in function or biomechanics exist.[4]

Diaphragm

Anatomically, the *diaphragm* is described as two separate muscles, the two portions differ in their functions. In 1978 Derenne et al.[4] were one of the first groups to describe the diaphragm's two actions, but were followed by a plethora of reports in the 1980s that supported this conclusion.[5,13,17,23–25]

Descriptions of the actions of the diaphragm and its component parts include models incorporating mechanical and pneumatic principles.[13,23] It is apparent that diaphragm muscle actions *cannot* be divorced from other components of the chest wall. The net result of contraction of the costal and/or crural portions depends on intercostal muscle activity, abdominal and pelvic floor muscle activity, and lung volumes, as well as other factors.[5,17,23] The complex integration of all these factors is discussed later in this chapter.

When the diaphragm contracts, abdominal pressure increases and pleural pressure decreases, resulting in an outward motion of the anterior chest wall and in lung inflation. The increased intra-abdominal pressure is also transmitted to the lower third of the rib cage at the zone of apposition, helping to push the lower ribs outward. As the dome of the diaphragm descends during contraction, abdominal contents are displaced caudally. Resistance to this displacement by the abdominal viscera, together with the increased abdominal pressures, fixes or anchors the diaphram dome. As the costal fibers continue to contract, the lower ribs are pulled upward.[4,17,24] The axis of rotation for the lower ribs is through the CV and CT joints, which are close to the sagittal plane, producing an increase in the lateral diameter of the thorax as the ribs are pulled upward.[5,26,27] This is the so-called bucket-handle motion of the lower ribs during inspiration. At low and normal lung volumes the costal diaphragm has a direct inspiratory action on the lower rib cage, even without increased abdominal pressure, and is considered to be in "series" (electrical model) with the crural diaphragm, intercostal muscles, and accessory muscles. The crural, which has no direct attachment to the rib cage, is in "parallel" with the intercostal and accessory muscles.[13,17,23]

Intercostals

Any discussion about the actions of the intercostals must include the parasternal and interosseous components of the internal, as well as external, intercostals. The controversy about the actions of the intercostal muscles dates back to the 18th century and continues today.[3,28–30] Hamberger's theory[3] of intercostal muscle actions is probably the most widely supported. His theory associated the actions of the three intercostal groups with their anatomic insertions and considered the axes of motion of the CV and CT joints. For example, the external intercostal, whose inferior insertion is farther from the ribs' axes of rotation than its superior insertion, causes greater torque to be produced on the lowermost rib by pulling it up further than the upper rib can be pulled downward. With such an action, the external intercostals would be considered inspiratory. The internal interosseous intercostals' contraction would have an opposite effect and be expiratory. The parasternal intercostals' proximal attachments are closely related to the sternum, so their actions are inspiratory.[29] The actions of the intercostal muscle groups just described have been observed electromyographically. These EMG studies, however, cannot distinguish among agonist, antagonist, synergist, and the stabilizing roles of muscle by using electrical activity.[28] Thus, the controversy continues.

Goldman and Mead's 1973 hypothesis[31] that the diaphragm is the only significant contracting muscle in quiet inspiration has been contradicted by several studies which demonstrate both EMG activity and shortening of the parasternals during quiet breathing.[5,31–33] Sampson and De Troyer[32] were able to demonstrate that the parasternal EMG activity during quiet breathing is not merely muscle spindle reflex activity. These authors also found that the parasternal internal and lateral (interosseous) external intercostal muscles, even in the same interspace, can act independently of each other, especially during loaded breathing.

When intercostal muscles, both internal and external, are stimulated, both ribs move toward each other, but the lower rib moves upward twice the distance that the upper rib moves downward. The ribs can be displaced more easily upward than downward, and compliance increases from the upper ribs to the lower ribs.[28] The rib elevating effect of the intercostal muscles is dependent on lung volume. At low lung volumes, intercostal muscle contraction results in a net elevation of the ribs, and at high lung volumes the effect is rib descent.[5,29] Sequencing of intercostal muscle contractions appear to occur in a cephalo-caudal direction during inspiration and in the opposite direction during expiration.[5,29] It appears that the external intercostals are more active during inspiration and the interosseous internal intercostals are more active during expiration, especially during active breathing, even though the intercostals intrinsically have the same mechanical activity.[5,29,34]

The above information about the actions and contributions of the intercostal muscle groups is not conclusive; the exact actions of these muscles are still not completely understood. Not mentioned are the possible contributions of other muscles which attach to the chest wall,[35] the possibility that the intercostals are more involved in postural motions of the thorax than ventilation,[5,29] and the possibility that some of the electrical activity measured in the intercostals is eccentric or antagonistic.[28] Future research needs to result from human studies in situ both at rest and under various conditions such as exercise and disease.

Scalenes

The scalenes are always active during inspiration, making them primary inspiratory muscles not accessory muscles. The scalenes, which attach to ribs 1 and 2, elevate the upper rib cage and the sternum. The action of the scalenes counteract the parasternals' tendency to pull the sternum downward. During quiet breathing, the scalenes must contract in coordination with the diaphragm and parasternals in upright humans for the rib cage to move with one degree of freedom (without distortion). During inspiration, as lung volume increases, the scalenes retain their contractile forces and mechanical efficiency.[5,19,25]

Accessory Muscles

The accessory muscles are not active during quiet breathing. They are extremely important during exercise, disease, forced breathing of any type, and unsupported upper extremity activities.[5,25]

Abdominals

The expiratory phase of quiet breathing is generally considered to be passive. The role of the abdominals in respiratory activities is often underestimated and relegated to coughing and other forced expiratory activities, including sneezing, defecation, and parturition. Abdominal muscles participate in both inspiration and expiration in addition to primarily functioning as rotators and flexors of the trunk.[2,4,5,36]

The rectus abdominus and external oblique muscles have been shown to act on the rib cage when they contract, whereas the internal oblique and transverse abdominus muscles do not appreciably move the rib cage when they are stimulated.[36] The rib cage deformation caused by the rectus and external obliques serve to decrease anterior-posterior and transverse diameters of the thorax, respectively.[5,37] In humans, isolated contraction of the rectus results in a small increase in the transverse rib cage diameter. These muscle contractions create two opposing actions on the transverse diameter of the thorax, but their net effect is to decrease rib cage diameter.

The abdominals also act to decrease lung volume by decreasing the antero-posterior diameter of the abdomen, thereby increasing intra-abdominal pressure, which displaces the diaphragm cranially, and increases pleural pressure. Paradoxically, the increased intra-abdominal pressure acts to push the lower ribs outward at the zone of opposition. Putting a stretch or increasing tension on the diaphragm would result in a pulling on the costal fibers to raise the lower ribs.[2,5]

The net effect of the opposing actions of the abdominals on the rib cage appears to depend on the balance between the muscle insertional forces (favoring expiration) and increasing abdominal pressure (favoring inspiration).[5,36] The tonic EMG activity in the abdominals, especially in the upright posture, helps to maintain a normal length–tension relationship of the diaphragm to maintain tidal volume (Vt).[5,38] Recruitment of abdominals occurs, especially at end-expiration, during exercise, CO_2 rebreathing, and in some disease states, such as chronic obstructive pulmonary disease (COPD).[2,5]

Triangularis Sterni

The actions of the TS have been recently studied in humans and found to be different from those in quadruped mammals, such as dogs and cats. It appears that the TS is not active, as are the abdominals during supine, tidal breathing. The TS is phasically active during quiet expiration and always active during expiratory maneuvers below functional residual capacity (FRC). The TS is activated along with the abdominals for active expiratory maneuvers (e.g., coughing, sneezing, talking, and singing) and for trunk movement and stabilization activities (e.g., trunk flexion and rotation and straight leg–raising).[5,22,32,39,40]

Quadratus Lumborum

The quadratus lumborum muscles contribute to ventilatory activities by stabilizing the lower rib pairs. This stabilization allows the crural diaphragm to eccentrically contract for coordinated and effective phonation.[9,21]

INTEGRATION AND COORDINATION OF THE VENTILATORY PUMP

The complexity of the integration and coordination of respiratory muscle activity and the resultant changes in chest wall configuration increase as a person changes position, exercises, performs other activities that involve the respiratory muscles, and develops various pulmonary and/or chest wall diseases or deformities. The respiratory control system is also complex and involves both automatic and voluntary regulation, receives input from a variety of receptors (chemoreceptors and mechanoreceptors), and can recruit numerous different groups of muscles for ventilation.[41] The actions of the ventilatory pump are designed to meet the metabolic demands of the body. The high level coordination of the respiratory muscles helps improve the efficiency of the system and may help prevent or delay ventilatory muscle fatigue.[41,42]

Goldman and Mead's theory[31] that during quiet inspiration the diaphragm is the only important contracting muscle has been disputed and found to be inaccurate. Coupling and coordination of the diaphragm and muscles that move the rib cage are necessary for the chest wall to move along its relaxation configuration.[5,19,43] From work by De Troyer and Estenne,[19] Sampson and De Troyer,[32] and others,[33,34] it is clear that the parasternal intercostals and the scalene muscles are primary muscles of inspiration. When V̇e requirement is large, there are extremely negative intrapleural pressures that work to collapse the thoracic cavity. The costal diaphragm helps to counteract this force for the lower rib cage, but the upper rib cage is protected by increased activity of the intercostal and neck accessory muscles.[41,43]

The activation of other ventilatory muscles not normally active during quiet inspiration is affected by habit, posture, and other simultaneous activities. As minute ventilation increases, ventilatory muscle recruitment increases.[2,43,44] Barnas et al.[45] studied chest wall impedances during a variety of nonrespiratory maneuvers. They concluded that a precise modulation of ventilatory and non-ventilatory muscles via mechanoreceptor feedback is necessary to continue breathing while sustaining contraction of ventilatory muscles involved in non-breathing activities.

The involvement of primary expiratory muscles in inspiratory activities has been described previously. The tonic abdominal muscle contraction effect that helps maintain the diaphragm in its optimal length–tension characteristic is dependent on posture. During quiet breathing it occurs only in the standing position.[5] The phasic effect of the abdominals which assists inspiration occurs in humans only during increased $\dot{V}e$ (e.g., during exercise). The abdominals contract during expiration, pushing the diaphragm cephalad and decreasing end-expiratory lung volume, so that when the abdominals relax at the end of expiration, lung volume will begin to increase before inspiration is actively under-way.[5,41]

The diaphragm is still the primary muscle of inspiration, and its actions, along with those of the other primary muscles of inspiration, produce a characteristic sequence of inspiratory chest wall motions during quiet breathing. Table 1-2 summarizes this usual sequence.

EFFECTS OF AGING ON THE VENTILATORY PUMP

The lungs, rib cage, and ventilatory muscles all change with normal growth and development. As humans develop from neonates to old age, the compliance, configuration, and mobility of the ventilatory pump changes. The changes in compliance of the rib cage and its articulations that occur with aging have major effects on ventilatory function. An infant's ribs are cartilaginous and therefore very compliant and easily distorted. "Super" compliant ribs, coupled with a more horizontal rib positioning, result in a primary stabilization function

Table 1-2. Sequence[a] of Chest Wall Motions During Quiet Inspiration

Motion	Explanation
1. Anterior abdominal wall pushed outward anteriorly	Descent of central tendon increases intra-abdominal pressure and displaces abdominal contents
2. Lower rib cage expands laterally	a. Costal fibers of diaphragm pull lower ribs upward b. Increased intra-abdominal pressures push lower ribs outward at zone of apposition
3. Upper rib cage expands anteriorly	Parasternal internal intercostal muscles and scalene muscles rotate upper ribs and elevate manubriosternum

[a] The motions described may occur in the sequence noted or simultaneously. Motion 3 often occurs simultaneously with motions 1 and 2. The extent of the motions observed also depends on body position.

of the chest wall muscles to counteract the diaphragm's tendency to pull the lower ribs inward.[46,47]

As age increases, chest wall compliance progressively decreases. Estenne et al.[48] measured chest wall compliance in adults ranging from 24 to 75 years old. They found statistically significant linear regression coefficients, demonstrating that as age increases, chest wall compliance decreases. Decreases in compliance were evident as early as the fourth decade. Ossification of the costal cartilages; fibrosis, fusion, and wear and tear of the chest wall articulations; general decreased muscle tone; and thoracic spine kyphosis all contribute to decreased chest wall compliance with advancing age.[49]

NORMAL ADAPTATIONS OF THE VENTILATORY PUMP TO PERTURBATIONS

As we all go about our normal activities of daily living, work, and play, we constantly alter the factors influencing the ventilatory pump. The perturbations of varying posture, changing lung volumes, and altering the mechanical load are naturally occurring events that influence $\dot{V}e$ and can be exacerbated by exercise and lung and chest wall disease and deformity.

Changes in Position or Posture

We are constantly changing body position throughout a 24-hour period. Sociocultural influences and habit significantly influence some of these changes and positions. The full range of effects of body position on functions of the pulmonary system is discussed in Chapter 5. This section reviews just some of the major known influences of posture on the ventilatory pump.

The direction of gravitational forces on the thorax and abdomen is altered upon changing body position. The interpretation of changes in respiratory muscles as posture is changed has been controversial[50] but is somewhat better understood today. As an individual moves from standing to sitting to supine, chest wall (rib cage) compliance and expiratory reserve volume (ERV) decrease due to the effect of gravity on the fluid-filled abdomen and the rib cage itself.[48,51] Diaphragm–abdomen compliance is higher in the supine position due to a decrease or elimination of intra-abdominal pressure against the anterior abdominal wall. Both insertional and appositional components of the diaphragm acting on the lower rib cage are reduced in supine,[48] but the diaphragm has a longer resting length and smaller curvature radius.[52] Many subjects recruit abdominal and TS muscles when upright, especially when breathing is increased (e.g., during exercise, CO_2 rebreathing), which optimizes diaphragmatic function.[52] It appears that the ventilatory muscles are able to nicely compensate and adjust to posture changes in normal, healthy persons under ordinary circumstances.

Changes in Volume

The changes in lung volume resulting from various respiratory maneuvers affect ventilatory pump function. The influence of lung volume on ventilatory muscle function is related to at least three major effects. The predominant effect is the influence of volume on the length–tension relationships of the various ventilatory muscles. The second major effect involves the effect of lung volume on sequential changes in compliance of the ribs and resulting intercostal muscle actions. The third effect, which involves only the diaphragm, is the loss of appositional intra-abdominal pressures.

Length–Tension and Volume

An important characteristic of skeletal muscle is that the force it can generate is dependent on its length. In 1978, Derenne et al.[4] noted that inspiratory muscles shorten and expiratory muscles lengthen during inspiration (and vice versa). These authors concluded that lung volume was therefore an index of respiratory muscle length. Dekhuijzen[53] notes that the parasternals' optimal resting lengths occur closer to total lung capacity (TLC). The diaphragm, which is primarily responsible for the generation of inspiratory forces (pressures), definitely shortens during inspiration and reaches its optimal resting length at FRC.[53,54] Although the radius of the diaphragm's curvature may also affect pressures generated during inspiration (Laplace's law), muscle fiber length is more important in determining diaphragmatic contractile forces.[55] The effects of lung volume on the intercostal muscles are more complicated, or at least more controversial, than those of the diaphragm. The intercostal muscles are included in discussions of length–tension effects of volume.

Intercostal Muscle Action Related to Lung Volume

Directional rib motion appears to be influenced directly by lung volume.[30] The interosseous portions of the internal and external intercostal muscles have similar effects on the ribs. The action of both internal and external intercostals at low lung volumes is to elevate the ribs. The effect is the opposite at high lung volumes. The explanation of these effects is complex, but a simplified version implies that the resistance to upward movement of the ribs is greater at high lung volumes (above neutral position) and that the ribs will therefore tend to be pulled down. Conversely, the relative compliance of the ribs is such that they are more easily moved upward at low lung volumes (rib cage below the neutral position).[30]

Changes in Appositional Abdominal Pressures on Rib Cage Motion

The inspiratory action of the diaphragm on rib cage motion has been described earlier in this chapter. When lung volumes decrease below FRC, the area of the rib cage apposed to the diaphragm is increased. This results in more opportunity for intra-abdominal pressure to push the lower rib cage outward. Conversely, at high lung volumes, the zone of apposition is decreased. At high lung volumes, intrapleural pressures can also tend to pull the rib cage inward. At TLC and in conditions of hyperaeration, the costal diaphragm fibers are no longer aligned vertically and tend to pull the lower ribs inward.[5]

Changes in Load

External and internal factors continually alter the loads on the ventilatory muscles even in normal, healthy individuals. Most factors that alter load, such as switching from mouth to nose breathing (doubles resistance to breathing), wearing restrictive clothing, and changing body position are naturally occurring.[8] Other phenomena that affect respiratory muscle loads include a person's state of consciousness and activity of other muscles.[50] Acute and chronic pulmonary disease and chest wall deformity and dysfunction can pathologically increase loads on the respiratory muscles by increasing airway resistance and decreasing chest wall and lung compliance. In addition, a disease such as COPD can change central inspiratory drive and length–tension relationships of the diaphragm.

The immediate response of the human respiratory system to an increase in mechanical load is a decrease in Vt, which gradually returns to normal levels if the load persists.[8] This is an example of how the respiratory system maintains $\dot{V}e$ as mechanical loads continually change. Load-compensation of the respiratory system helps to maintain ventilatory stability. The mechanisms involved in load-compensation include chemoreceptor–central nervous system control, pulmonary receptor reflexes (e.g., Hering-Breuer reflex), mechanoreceptor reflexes, respiratory muscle proprioception, force–length and force–velocity relationships of the respiratory muscles, mechanical arrangement of the respiratory muscles, and the biomechanics of the thorax.[4,8,32,50] The ventilatory responses to changes in load may depend on consciousness and may be subject to learned patterns.[8]

Conformational changes in the rib cage have been noted by several investigators.[32,56] Sampson and De Troyer[32] compared rib cage distortion between elastic and resistive loads and found no differences. These authors found also that rib cage distortion patterns depends on which respiratory muscles are active during the loaded breathing, and that there is much individual variability. All subjects showed increases in lateral diameter of their rib cages and increased EMG activity in the lateral intercostal muscles. A few subjects also had increases in anteroposterior diameter of their rib cages associated with increased activity in the parasternal intercostal muscles.[32] Distortion of the rib cage during loaded breathing may be further influenced by the level of fatigue of the inspiratory muscles. Paradoxic and asynchronous rib cage motions have been observed in subjects just before and during respiratory muscle fatigue.[57]

Chronic, persistent loading of the ventilatory pump can occur in situations such as obesity, pulmonary disease, and thoracic deformity. A recent study by Tarasiuk et al.[58] examined the effects of five weeks' chronic resistive loading (using a tracheal cannula) on respiratory muscle mass, composition, and contractile performance in rats. These authors found that respiratory muscle composition and function change with chronic loading and that the responses of the diaphragm and the SCM muscles were different. Further study is needed to better understand the differences in adaptive changes of the ventilatory muscles.

SUMMARY

This chapter reviewed the current literature and described the structure and function of the ventilatory pump as we understand it today. The complexity of the control of $\dot{V}e$ and of the responses of the ventilatory pump to natural and pathologic influences is in contrast to its relatively simple structure. The ventilatory muscles, and the ventilatory pump in general, are unique compared to other skeletal muscles because they must contract continuously throughout life; their control is both voluntary and involuntary; and they work against elastic (chest wall and lungs) and resistive (airways) loads rather than against gravity.[4,59] These unique characteristics, together with the fact that ventilatory muscles function in activities other than $\dot{V}e$, result in a fascinating area for kinesiologic and biomechanic investigation. There are so many aspects of ventilatory physiology that are unknown or not clearly understood. As technology improves, our ability to define some of these aspects also improve, but it is still difficult to identify specific actions of various ventilatory muscles in natural breathing situations in human subjects. It is hoped that many of the questions about ventilatory physiology will soon be answered, and that our increased understanding of the normal structure and functions of ventilation will enable health care professionals to better evaluate and treat patients with respiratory system disease and dysfunction.

REFERENCES

1. Wasserman K, Whipp BJ: State of the art: exercise physiology in health and disease. Am Rev Respir Dis 112:219, 1975
2. Celli BR: Clinical and physiologic evaluation of respiratory muscle function. Clin Chest Med 10:199, 1989

3. Hamberger GE: De respirationis mechanismo et usu genuino. Iena, Germany, 1749
4. Derenne JPH, Macklem PT, and Roussos CH: State of the art: the respiratory muscles: mechanics, control and pathophysiology (part 1). Am Rev Respir Dis 118:119, 1978
5. De Troyer A, Estenne M: Functional anatomy of the respiratory muscles. Clin Chest Med 9:175, 1988
6. Bouhuys A: The Physiology of Breathing. Grune & Stratton, Orlando, FL, 1977
7. Davis GM, Bureau MA: Pulmonary and chest wall mechanics in the control of respiration in the newborn. Clin Perinatol 14:551, 1987
8. Campbell EJM, Agostini E, Davis JN: The Respiratory Muscles: Mechanics and Neural Control. WB Saunders, Philadelphia, 1970
9. Schaefer RC: Clinical Biomechanics: Musculoskeletal Actions and Reactions. Williams & Wilkins, Baltimore, 1983
10. Fam AG, Smythe HA: Musculoskeletal chest wall pain. Can Med Assoc J 133:379, 1985
11. Pick TP, Howden R (eds): Gray's Anatomy. Running Press, Philadelphia, 1974
12. Panicek DM, Benson CB, Gottlieb RH et al: The diaphragm: anatomic, pathologic and radiologic considerations. Radiographics 8:385, 1988
13. De Troyer A, Sampson MG, Sigrist S, Macklem PT: The diaphragm: two muscles. Science 213:237, 1981
14. Supinski GS: Respiratory muscle blood supply. Clin Chest Med 9:211, 1988
15. Belman MJ, Sieck GC: The ventilatory muscles: fatigue, endurance and training. Chest 82:761, 1982
16. Faulkner JA, Maxwell LC, Roff GL, White TP: The diaphragm as a muscle: contractile properties (part 2). Am Rev Respir Dis 119:89, 1979
17. Rochester DF: The diaphragm: contractile properties and fatigue. J Clin Invest 75:1397, 1985
18. Sharp JT: Therapeutic considerations in respiratory muscle function. Chest suppl. 88:S118, 1985
19. De Troyer A, Estenne M: Coordination of rib cage muscles and diaphragm during quiet breathing in humans. J Appl Physiol 57:899, 1984
20. Quiring DP, Warfel JH: The Head, Neck and Trunk: Muscles and Motor Points. Lea & Febiger. Philadelphia, 1967
21. Basmajian JV, DeLuca CJ: Muscles Alive. 5th Ed. Williams & Wilkins, Baltimore, 1985
22. De Troyer A, Ninane V, Gilmartin JJ et al: Triangularis sterni muscle use in supine humans. J Appl Physiol 62:919, 1987
23. Kapandji IA: The Physiology of the Joints. Churchill Livingstone, Edinburgh, 1974
24. Sharp JT, Goldberg NB, Druz WS et al: Relative contributions of rib cage and abdomen to breathing in normal subjects. J Appl Physiol 39:608, 1975
25. Macklem PT, Macklem DM, De Troyer A: A model of inspiratory muscle mechanics. J Appl Physiol 55:547, 1983
26. Roussos CH, Macklem PT: The respiratory muscles. N Engl J Med 307:786, 1982
27. Celli BR: Respiratory muscle function. Clin Chest Med 7:567, 1986
28. Wilson TA, Rehder K, Krayer S et al: Geometry and respiratory displacement of human ribs. J Appl Physiol 62:1872, 1987
29. De Troyer A, Kelly S, Zin WA: Mechanical action of the intercostal muscles on the ribs. Science 220:87, 1983
30. De Troyer A, Kelly S, Macklem PT, Zin WA: Mechanics of intercostal space and actions of external and internal intercostal muscles. J Clin Invest 75:850, 1985

31. Goldman MD, Mead J: Mechanical interaction between the diaphragm and rib cage. J Appl Physiol 35:197, 1973
32. Sampson MG, De Troyer A: Role of intercostal muscles in the rib cage distortions produced by inspiratory loads. J Appl Physiol 52:517, 1982
33. Taylor A: The contribution of intercostal muscles to the effort of respiration in man. J Physiol (Lond) 151:390, 1960
34. De Troyer A, Sampson MG: Activation of the parasternal intercostals during breathing efforts in human subjects. J Appl Physiol 52:524, 1982
35. Saumerez RC: An analysis of action of intercostal muscles in human upper rib cage. J Appl Physiol 60:690, 1986
36. De Troyer A, Farkas GA: Mechanical arrangement of the parasternal intercostals in the different interspaces. J Appl Physiol 66:1421, 1989
37. De Troyer A, Sampson MG, Sigrist S, Kelly S: How the abdominal muscles act on the rib cage. J Appl Physiol 54:465, 1983
38. Mier A, Brophy C, Estenne M et al: Action of abdominal muscles on rib cage in humans. J Appl Physiol 58:1438, 1985
39. Strohl KP, Mead J, Banzett RB et al: Effect of posture on upper and lower rib cage motion and tidal volume during diaphragm pacing. Am Rev Respir Dis 130:320, 1984
40. Estenne M, Ninane V, De Troyer A: Triangularis sterni muscle use during eupnea in humans: effect of posture. Resp Physiol 74:151, 1988
41. Cherniack NS: The central nervous system and respiratory muscle coordination. Chest suppl. 97:S52, 1990
42. Roussos CH, Moxam J: Respiratory muscle fatigue. p. 829. In: Roussos CH, Macklem PT (eds): Thorax. New York, Marcel Dekker, 1985
43. Rochester DF: Respiratory muscle function in health. Heart and Lung 13:349, 1984
44. Kim MJ, Larson JL: Ineffective airway clearance and ineffective breathing patterns: theoretical and research base for nursing diagnosis. Nurs Clin North Am 22:125, 1987
45. Barnas GM, Mills PJ, Mackenzie CF et al: Regional chest wall impedance during nonrespiratory maneuvers. J Appl Physiol 70:42, 1991
46. Davis GM, Bureau MA: Pulmonary and chest wall biomechanics in the control of respiration in the newborn. Clin Perinatol 14:551, 1987
47. Crane LD: The thorax and chest wall. p. 178. In: Norkin C, Levange P (eds): Joint Structure and Function. 2nd Ed. FA Davis, Philadelphia, 1992
48. Estenne M, Yernault JC, De Troyer A: Rib cage and diaphragm-abdomen compliance in humans: effects of age and posture. J Appl Physiol 59:1842, 1985
49. Krumpe PE, Knudson RJ, Parsons G, Reiser K: The aging respiratory system. Clin Geriatr Med 1:143, 1985
50. Derenne JPH, Macklem PT, Roussos CH: State of the art: the respiratory muscles Mechanics, control and pathophysiology (part 2). Am Rev Respir Dis 118:373, 1978
51. Peters RM: The mechanical basis of respiration. Boston Little, Brown & Co, 1969
52. Lopata M, O'Conner TD, Onal E: Effects of position on respiratory muscle function during CO_2 rebreathing. Respiration 47:98, 1985
53. Dekhuijzen PNR: Target-flow inspiratory muscle training and pulmonary rehabilitation in patients with chronic obstructive pulmonary disease. Thesis, Department of Pulmonary Diseases, University of Nijmegen, Medical Centre Dekkerswald, Groesbeek, The Netherlands, 1989
54. Tobin MJ: Respiratory muscles in disease. Clin Chest Med 9:263, 1988
55. Kim MJ: Druz WS, Danan J et al: Mechanics of the canine diaphragm. J Appl Physiol 41:369, 1976

56. Agostoni E, Magnoni P: Deformation of the chest wall during breathing efforts. J Appl Physiol 21:1827, 1966
57. Rochester DF: Tests of respiratory muscle function. Clin Chest Med 9:249, 1988
58. Tarasiuk A, Scharf SM, Miller MJ: Effect of chronic resistive loading on inspiratory muscles in rats. J Appl Physiol 70:216, 1991
59. Rochester DF, Braun NM: The respiratory muscles. Basics Resp Dis 6:1, 1978

2 | Cardiopulmonary Response to Exercise

Scot Irwin
Cynthia Coffin Zadai

Although there is a rapidly evolving body of literature on the pulmonary response to exercise, a discussion about the pulmonary system independent from the cardiac system would create a void in the understanding of the complex and interrelated oxygen transport system. The primary focus of this chapter is the normal cardiac and pulmonary responses to exercise, illustrating both similarities and differences between the systems, so as to establish a basic understanding of the normal mechanics of oxygen transport in relation to exercise demands. This groundwork is used in subsequent chapters to explore the abnormal responses seen in the clinical setting, thereby assisting the clinician in identifying each client's individual limitations and establishing the primary focus for therapeutic intervention.

The basic formula for describing oxygen uptake is expressed as follows: $\dot{V}O_2 = (\dot{Q}) \times (a - \bar{v}O_2 \text{ diff})$. This formula is defined as the volume of oxygen consumed ($\dot{V}O_2$) is equal to the cardiac output ($\dot{Q}$) multiplied by the arterial oxygen content (a) minus the central venous ($\bar{v}$) oxygen content (O_2) difference (diff). The higher an individual's $\dot{V}O_2$ max, the higher the level of cardiopulmonary fitness. Ventilation ($\dot{V}e$) and $\dot{Q}$ are the key components that contribute to delivering the oxygen necessary to achieve a desired level of exercise.

VENTILATORY RESPONSE TO EXERCISE

Ventilation

Ventilation is equal to the respiratory rate (RR) times the tidal volume (Vt) and is curvalinearly related to an individual's maximum oxygen consumption

23

(Fig. 2-1). Maximum ventilation ($\dot{V}e$ max) in liters per minute is linearly related to maximum oxygen uptake ($\dot{V}O_2$ max) (Fig. 2-2).

Resting values for $\dot{V}e$, RR, and Vt are well known and not significantly different between individuals when adjusted by anthropometric measurements for sex and age. Normal adult values for $\dot{V}e$ range from 6.0 to 10.0 L/min at rest produced by a Vt of 400 to 850 ml per breath and a respiratory rate of 10 to 20 breaths per minute. Maximum exercise values for the adult range from 100 to

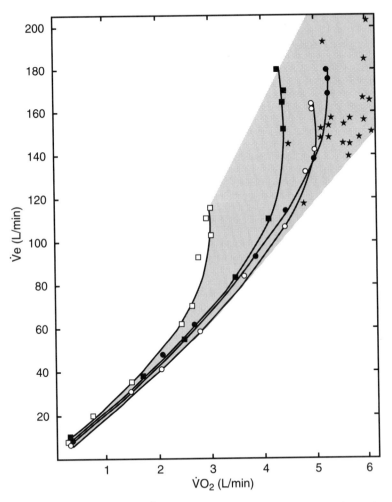

Fig. 2-1. Pulmonary ventilation ($\dot{V}e$) at rest and during exercise (running or cycling). Four individual curves are presented. Several rates of exercise gave the same maximal oxygen uptake ($\dot{V}O_2$ max). Exercise time is from 2 to 6 minutes. Stars denote individual values for top athletes measured when $\dot{V}O_2$ max was obtained. Individuals with $\dot{V}O_2$ max of 3 L/min or higher usually fall within the shadowed area. Note the wide scattering at high $\dot{V}O_2$. (From Åstrand and Rodahl,[1] with permission.)

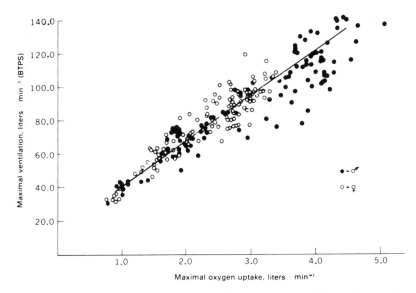

Fig. 2-2. Data on 225 subjects from 4 to about 30 years old: maximal pulmonary ventilation ($\dot{V}e$ max) in relation to maximal oxygen uptake ($\dot{V}O_2$ max) measured during running on a motor-driven treadmill for about 5 minutes. (From Åstrand and Rodahl,[1] with permission.)

200 L/min on average and can go up to 200 L/min for world-class athletes. The mean values for maximum tidal volume ($\bar{V}t$ max) of exercising males is 2.7 to 2.9 L/min and 1.9 to 2.7 L/min in females. Maximum RR during exercise is 40 to 50 breaths per minute for both sexes.[1,2,3]

Recently, Blackie et al.[3] studied and recorded mean values and ranges for ventilatory responses ($\dot{V}e$, RR, Vt) during maximal exercise in healthy men and women 20 to 80 years of age. Each decade of age was grouped separately and each had 20 subjects, with the exception of the 70- to 79-year-old males, which numbered 11. Data were collected from 231 normal subjects (120 women and 111 men) who each performed a maximum symptom-limited exercise test on a bicycle ergometer. The mean values for ventilatory responses are found in Table 2-1. The authors concluded that mean maximum ventilation ($\bar{V}e$ max) was significantly lower for women than men across all age groups. The primary variable causing this difference was Vt, as RR max were not significantly different.[3]

Secondly, age decremental losses in ventilatory ability appeared to be minimal up to the sixth decade. Major decrements appeared in the sixth and seventh decades, but there was wide variation among individual responses. The study also demonstrated that mean maximum voluntary ventilation (MVV) was 61 percent $\bar{V}e$ max during exercise. This is similar to findings of several other studies,[1,2,4–7] but the authors are quick to point out the wide range of differences in each individual's ability to utilize a percentage of the MVV. One subject

Table 2-1. Mean Values for Ventilation at End of Exercise[a]

Group and Age (Years)	V̇e max (L/min)	RR max (Breaths/min)	Vt max (L)	V̇e max/MVV
Men				
20–29	114 ± 23	42 ± 8	2.7 ± 0.4	0.63 ± 0.10
30–39	105 ± 30	40 ± 15	2.7 ± 0.6	0.62 ± 0.19
40–49	102 ± 23	36 ± 7	2.9 ± 0.6	0.63 ± 0.14
50–59	97 ± 15	36 ± 6	2.8 ± 0.3	0.66 ± 0.13
60–69	83 ± 14	33 ± 6	2.6 ± 0.4	0.61 ± 0.12
70–79	66 ± 12	30 ± 6	2.3 ± 0.4	0.54 ± 0.09
Mean ± SD	97 ± 25	36 ± 9	2.7 ± 0.5	0.62 ± 0.14
Women				
20–29	87 ± 17	41 ± 7	2.2 ± 0.5	0.61 ± 0.09
30–39	88 ± 19	44 ± 8	2.0 ± 0.3	0.66 ± 0.13
40–49	74 ± 15	35 ± 8	2.1 ± 0.4	0.57 ± 0.13
50–59	60 ± 15	32 ± 8	1.9 ± 0.4	0.58 ± 0.16
60–69	56 ± 14	33 ± 9	1.7 ± 0.2	0.57 ± 0.17
70–79	48 ± 12	31 ± 7	1.6 ± 0.3	0.56 ± 0.14
Mean ± SD	69 ± 22	36 ± 9	1.9 ± 0.4	0.59 ± 0.14

Abbreviations: V̇e max, maximum ventilation; RR max, maximum respiratory rate; breaths/min, breaths per minute; Vt max, maximum tidal volume; MVV, maximum voluntary ventilation.
[a] Note that $N = 20$ for each age group except men aged 70 to 79 years (where $N = 11$).
(From Blackie et al.,[3] with permission.)

actually exceeded his MVV during exercise, while several others were able to utilize only 40 percent of MVV. This wide variability is depicted in Figure 2-3.

Finally, Blackie et al. found that the range of breathing patterns used during exercise was quite variable within the normal healthy population and that the best correlates with maximum ventilation (V̇e max) were maximum carbon dioxide production (V̇CO_2 max) and V̇O_2 max.[3] Other resting static lung volumes—forced vital capacity (FVC), forced expiratory volume in one second (FEV_1), and tidal volume–to–FVC ratio—correlated with V̇e max values but were not as significantly strong correlates as V̇CO_2 and V̇O_2 maximums.[3]

The ventilatory response to exertion in the normal untrained individual is fairly reproducible and best illustrated graphically. Figure 2-4 depicts the normal relationship between RR and Vt as an individual works from rest to V̇O_2 max.[2] This relationship is most easily described as a rate-to-volume synchronization. At low levels of exercise (less than 50 percent of V̇O_2 max), an individual is most dependent upon increases in Vt to increase total V̇e. Once the level of exercise exceeds 50 percent of an individual's V̇O_2 max, the primary contribution to increases in V̇e is a result of an increase in the frequency of breathing. In fact, the Vt or depth of breathing commonly levels off at 50 percent of an individual's vital capacity (VC). This relationship between Vt max and FVC is shown in Figure 2-5.

The point where V̇e becomes nonlinear in its relationship to oxygen consumption is referred to as the ventilatory threshold[1] (Fig. 2-1). There appears to be a relationship between this point and the onset of measurable lactate levels in the venous blood.[8] Recently, there has been some controversy in the literature

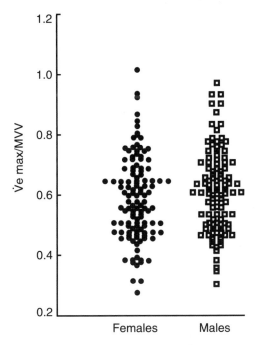

Fig. 2-3. Range of values for maximal ventilation (V̇e max) corrected for maximal voluntary ventilation (MVV) at end of exercise. Each point represents an individual subject. (From Blackie et al.,[3] with permission.)

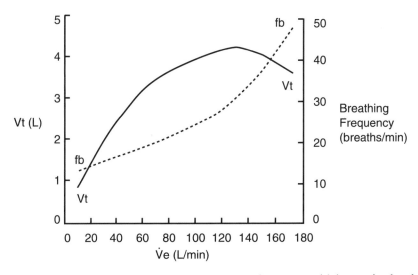

Fig. 2-4. Changes in tidal volume (Vt) and breathing frequency with increasing levels of ventilation (V̇e) in exercise. (From Pardy et al.,[2] with permission.)

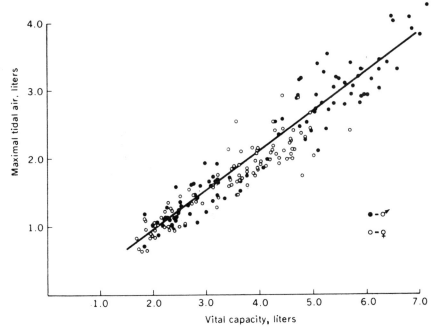

Fig. 2-5. Highest tidal volume (Vt max) measured during running at submaximal and maximal speed (exercise time about 5 minutes) related to the individual's vital capacity (VC) measured in standing position. Altogether, 190 subjects, from 7 to 30 years old, are shown. On average, 50 to 55 percent of the VC is used as Vt max. (From Åstrand and Rodahl,[1] with permission.)

regarding the significance of this relationship, as disparity has been found between the onset of the lactate or so-called anaerobic threshold and the ventilatory threshold. In individuals who are using a rapid pedaling speed,[9] have previously exercised,[10] or have ingested caffeine,[11] there has been a lack of correlation between lactate levels and change in V̇e.

Over the last decade and a half, a plethora of scientific articles have developed and promoted the concept of an anaerobic threshold.[8,10-15] As first described by Wasserman et al.,[8] the anaerobic threshold is defined as the work rate or V̇O$_2$ beyond which measurable levels of lactic acid begin to accumulate in the blood, indicating achievement of an increased reliance on anaerobic energy sources. Their original investigation found that this increase in lactic acid was closely associated with a nonlinear increase in V̇e. Since their initial discovery, though, several additions and refinements of the concept have appeared in the literature. The terminology most commonly used currently to describe these threshold phenomena are the lactate threshold[10] and the ventilatory threshold.[11]

Use of the term *anaerobic threshold,* or even *lactate threshold,* has some inherent problems. First, the student of exercise physiology needs to recognize that anaerobic metabolism is an integral part of energy production at all levels of exercise and not strictly limited to exercise that exceeds 50 percent of an individual's $\dot{V}O_2$ max. Second, the parameters for identifying the amount of lactate accumulation required to signify an individual's threshold varies from individual to individual. Finally, measurement and use of the anaerobic threshold as a clinical indicator is difficult, costly, and of questionable clinical relevance.

What are the limits to $\dot{V}e$ max? As we have already noted, Vt max during exercise is limited to approximately 50 percent of an individual's VC. The maximum breathing rate appears to be around 40 to 50 breaths per minute. The physiologic reasons for these maximum limits are not clear. Higher values can be achieved by normal individuals at rest during volitional effort. Some individuals cannot approach mean normal values due to abnormal chest wall mechanics, pathologic lung processes, or limitations of musculoskeletal function. In others, such as world-class athletes, these predicted maximum values can be exceeded.

Why are some individuals able to use a greater percentage of their MVV during maximum exercise than others? Why don't individuals achieve an exercise $\dot{V}e$ max equal to their MVV? Perhaps the contribution of the accessory muscles of ventilation to the activity being performed (e.g., rowing, biking) limits the musculoskeletal pump's total ability to participate in ventilation. For example, the contributions of the abdominal musculature to stabilization of the pelvis during running or even fast walking may be sufficient to limit their participation in active expiration, especially at maximum levels of exercise.

Gas Exchange

How does an individual's ventilatory ability relate to the formula, $\dot{V}O_2 = (\dot{Q}) \times (a - \bar{v}O_2 \text{ diff})$? Ventilation is required to maintain the arterial oxygen content and to eliminate carbon dioxide. Oxygen is extracted from the atmosphere and gradually achieves a partial pressure in the arterial system (PaO_2) of 90 to 100 mmHg in normal individuals. Figure 2-6 shows the pressure changes of oxygen that occur from the atmosphere, where the partial pressure is about 159 mmHg at sea level, to the PaO_2. This pressure change is dependent on adequate gas mixing, surface area for diffusion, driving pressure of oxygen between the alveolus and the capillary, and the lack of diffusion barriers.

The PaO_2 is directly related to the oxygen content of arterial blood. This relationship is expressed by the oxyhemoglobin disassociation curve (Fig. 2-7). The oxygen-carrying capacity of arterial blood is expressed by the following equation: 1.34 ml of O_2 per gram of hemoglobin times the number of grams of hemoglobin per 100 ml of blood, times the percent saturation of the hemoglobin. When expressed mathematically, using the average male hemoglobin level of 15 g pr 100 ml of blood and a percent saturation of 97 percent, the formula looks like this: (1.34 ml $O_2 \times 15$ gHg) (.97) = an O_2 content of 20.1 vol %. This is the oxygen-carrying capacity of arterial blood that is 97 percent saturated with oxygen. In the $\dot{V}O_2$ equation, this would be equal to the oxygen content of the

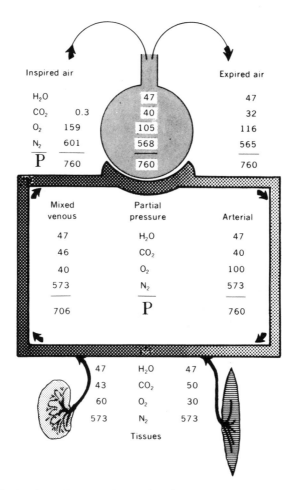

Fig. 2-6. Typical values of gas tensions in inspired air, alveolar air (encircled), expired air, and blood, at rest. Barometric pressure = 760 mmHg (100 mmHg = kPa). For simplicity, the inspired air is considered free from water (dry). Tension of O_2 and CO_2 varies markedly in venous blood from different organs. In this figure, gas tensions in venous blood from the kidney and muscle are presented. (From Åstrand and Rodahl,[1] with permission.)

arterial blood, or the small *a* in (a − $\bar{v}O_2$ diff). The $\bar{v}O_2$ content is determined by the same formula and is significantly lower because the saturation of venous blood is decreased. The decrease is a result of the working muscle or organ extracting the oxygen to create adenosine triphosphate (ATP) and thereby reduces the blood's oxygen content.

Any time the PaO_2 drops, the oxygen saturation of the blood decreases. This is not a linear phenomena, as can be seen in Figure 2-7A. The physiologic

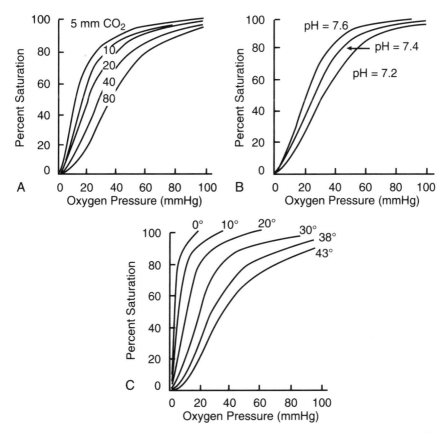

Fig. 2-7. Effects of **(A)** CO_2, **(B)** pH, and **(C)** temperature (°C) on the oxygen disso-ciation curve of the blood. Percent of saturation = percent HbO_2. (From Åstrand and Rodahl,[1] with permission.)

reason for the curvilinear relationship is created by the molecular affinity of oxygen for hemoglobin, which becomes more tenacious as the oxygen content of hemoglobin decreases. When the PaO_2 decreases and the saturation of hemo-globin decreases, the affinity of oxygen for hemoglobin increases. There are numerous factors that affect the slope and character of this curve. For example, when the pH of blood decreases, the curve shifts to the right (Fig. 2-7B). When the temperature at the tissue level increases, the curve also shifts to the right (Fig. 2-7C). Shifts to the right cause an improvement in oxygen delivery at the tissue level because the increase in temperature and acidity tend to reduce the affinity of oxygen for hemoglobin even at low saturation levels. This is very advantageous to the exercising individual, as tissue temperature and pH are elevated and decreased respectively, enhancing oxygen delivery to the tissues.

    In the normal untrained person, the PaO_2 rarely falls even during extremes of exercise. However, there is some evidence to indicate that the well-trained athlete may not maintain PaO_2 and saturation during maximum levels of exercise.[16] One theory proposed to explain this phenomena is that these individuals have sufficient $\dot{Q}$ to increase $\dot{V}O_2$ and delivery, but the majority or even all of the additional oxygen taken in is consumed by the ventilatory muscles.[16] In effect, the ventilatory muscles steal away the increases in $\dot{V}O_2$ from the muscles performing a task.

As the demand for oxygen increases, the pulmonary $\dot{V}e$ rises. There is in turn an oxygen cost for the work performed by the respiratory muscles to meet the increased ventilatory requirements. This oxygen demand is expressed as the number of liters of air required per liter of O_2 consumed. In healthy adults at low levels of exercise, this ratio is 20 to 25 L of air per liter of $\dot{V}O_2$.[1] This relationship varies with even moderate levels of exercise, but with high levels of exercise, the cost increases to 30 to 40 L of air per liter of $\dot{V}O_2$ required. At rest, the ventilatory muscles use 0.5 to 1.0 ml of O_2 per liter of $\dot{V}e$. This is less than 1 percent of the total $\dot{V}O_2$. As $\dot{V}e$ increases, the O_2 cost per liter of $\dot{V}e$ increases. During extremes of exercise, up to 10 percent of the total $\dot{V}O_2$ may be required to fuel the muscles of respiration. Pardy et al.[2] found that at $\dot{V}e$ levels above 130 L/min, there was a steep rise in the oxygen cost for work performed by the ventilatory muscles (or the work of breathing [WOB]).[2] In fact, Otis[17] estimated that at ventilations in excess of 140 L/min, all increases in oxygen uptake would be totally consumed by the ventilatory muscles.[17] Simultaneously, the muscles of ventilation must also receive a significant portion of the $\dot{Q}$. During exercise requiring a ventilatory volume of 130 to 180 L/min, 15 to 25 percent of the total $\dot{Q}$ may be going to the respiratory muscles. Obviously, this leaves a significantly smaller portion of the $\dot{Q}$ supply available to the other working muscles. The relationship among $\dot{V}O_2$, $\dot{Q}$, $\dot{V}e$, and the oxygen cost of $\dot{V}e$ further enforces the need for the clinician to observe and measure both the cardiac and pulmonary responses during exercise in order to determine the true limitations to each client's ability to perform work.

The previous discussion gives some support to the concept that $\dot{V}e$, not $\dot{Q}$ may be the limiting factor to maximum exercise. The case for $\dot{Q}$, though, is very strong. There is a wealth of data establishing maximum $\dot{Q}$ as the primary limitation to increase in $\dot{V}O_2$ max in normal adults.[1] This is primarily true because $\dot{V}e$ max can be artificially increased even at maximum levels of exercise. There is one study which puts the question in doubt. When Brice and Welch[18] substituted 79 percent helium and 21 percent oxygen for air, the reduction in mixture density and thus airflow resistance allowed for a significant increase in both $\dot{V}e$ max and $\dot{V}O_2$.[18] However, since $\dot{V}e$ cannot be conclusively established as the limiting factor in the $\dot{V}O_2$ max of normal adults, $\dot{Q}$ must be considered as the most likely alternative.

CARDIAC RESPONSES TO EXERCISE

Cardiac output is the next portion of the $\dot{V}O_2$ formula requiring discussion. $\dot{Q}$ is equal to the heart rate (HR) multiplied by the stroke volume (SV), or: $\dot{Q} = HR \times SV$). The progression of the normal adult HR response from rest to maximum exercise is primarily a linear process directly related to increase in $\dot{V}O_2$ (Fig. 2-8). At extreme levels of exercise intensity, the HR response becomes mildly curvilinear. In contrast, SV response to exercise is much the same as the Vt response. The majority of SV change occurs during low to moderate levels of exercise and then levels off at approximately 50 percent of $\dot{V}O_2$ max (Fig. 2-8). The normal healthy adult can achieve a maximum HR approaching the result of the formula 220 − age. This formula does not take into account the wide variation in maximum HR between individuals caused by their state of fitness, disease, or other environmental factors that can affect heart rate.

Maximum $\dot{Q}$ is primarily influenced by maximum SV. Increases in $\dot{Q}$ are directly and linearly related to increases in $\dot{V}O_2$ max. Thus, the factors which most directly affect SV have the most profound effects on $\dot{V}O_2$ max. SV is a function of venous return, peripheral vascular resistance, and myocardial contractility and distensibility. Distensibility is a function of the degree to which diastolic filling can be increased without expanding the ventricles beyond optimal contractile length. SV can be effectively modified by a change in any one of these factors. If, for example, an individual changes body position form supine, where venous return is facilitated, to sitting or standing, SV is decreased momentarily until the same level of venous return can be reestablished.

SV should increase with the onset of exercise, due to advantageous alteration of each of the physiologic factors mentioned. Venous return is enhanced by the onset of lower extremity muscular contraction, while myocardial contrac-

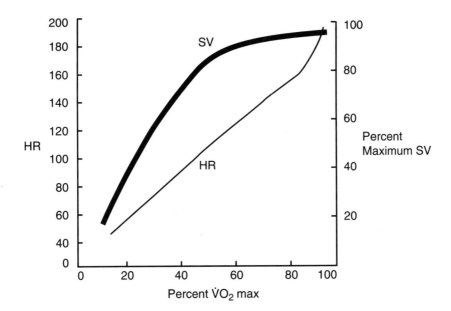

Fig. 2-8. Heart rate (HR) and stroke volume (SV) response in relation to percentage of maximum oxygen uptake.

tility improves with sympathetic stimulation and stretch of the cardiac muscle (Frank-Starling mechanism). Peripheral vascular resistance on the arterial side is also reduced initially during exercise due to vasodilatation of the arterioles. All of these factors work together to improve SV and thus increase cardiac output, which directly enhances $\dot{V}O_2$.

EVALUATION OF CARDIAC RESPONSES

Patients with chronic hypoxia, hypercapnia, and poor pulmonary function may have a multitude of factors that limit exercise tolerance. Physiologic factors limiting performance may include increased WOB due to airflow obstruction or poor chest wall mechanics, diaphragmatic dysfunction due to paralysis or years of deconditioning, and increased resistance to airflow. All of the pulmonary (ventilatory and gas exchange) limitations will be discussed in Chapter 3. However, the cardiac limitations to exercise in patients with pulmonary disease may often be overlooked, especially within the milieu of abnormal blood gases or pulmonary function tests and patient complaints of dyspnea. Clinically, cardiac dysfunction, especially right ventricular dysfunction, may prove to be the major limitation to increase in $\dot{V}O_2$ and thus exercise tolerance in patients with pulmonary disease.[19,20]

A study of Morrison et al.[20] found a strong correlation between right ventricular function as measured by ejection fraction and $\dot{V}O_2$ in patients with chronic obstructive pulmonary disease (COPD). At the same time, they found very poor correlations with resting PaO_2 (r = .29), exercise PaO_2 (r = .12), resting and exercise O_2 content (r = .21), or FEV_1 (r = .19) and $\dot{V}O_2$ overall. Total $\dot{V}e$ was highly correlated with $\dot{V}O_2$, but as already discussed, this is true in normal individuals as well. The authors also noted that their subjects demonstrated only small increases in $PaCO_2$ during exercise and 7 of their 25 subjects demonstrated no significant increase. The overall conclusion drawn by the investigators was that a major contribution to the limited $\dot{V}O_2$ seen in the COPD population is dysfunction of the right ventricle.[19] A key finding in this and other studies was the abnormal increase in pulmonary artery pressure which occurred with exercise.[21,22] This is just the opposite of the normal response, which is a decline in pulmonary vascular resistance with exercise.[23]

There are several potential causes for right ventricular dysfunction in patients with COPD: (1) loss of lung parenchyma reduces the cross-sectional area of the pulmonary capillary bed; (2) polycythemia and abnormal sodium secretion result in hypervolemia; (3) poor ventilatory mechanics and high intrathoracic pressures impair venous return; and (4) air trapping in the lower lobes may compress pulmonary vessels.

Obviously, there are many factors that impact upon the $\dot{V}O_2$ max of patients with COPD. The mechanism responsible for exercise limitation is probably an interplay of several factors, including efficiency of gas exchange, ventilatory mechanics, and $\dot{Q}$ (see Ch. 3). The clinician may be able to identify $\dot{Q}$ as a limitation to exercise by carefully monitoring the patient's blood pressure response at rest and with activity. The normal blood pressure response to exercise is to have a moderate rise in blood pressure with increasing levels of exercise and HR. A fall in systolic pressure or a flat blood pressure response with a concomitant increase in HR may signify cardiac dysfunction. In the patient population with COPD, this is potentially a result of right ventricular dysfunction.

SUMMARY

This chapter has reviewed the normal cardiac and pulmonary response to exercise. There is a wide variation in the breathing patterns selected by individuals in response to the increased oxygen demand of exercise from initiation to maximal levels. However, the correlation between $\dot{V}e$ and $\dot{Q}$ to $\dot{V}O_2$ max is strong. The formula for measuring $\dot{V}O_2$ directs the clinician when analyzing the adequacy of each component of the cardiopulmonary system's capacity to achieve $\dot{V}O_2$ max. The combination of $\dot{V}e$ and $\dot{Q}$ is required to meet any increased demand for $\dot{V}O_2$, and each of these systems has a myriad of variables that can effect each system's ability to participate in achieving the desired $\dot{V}O_2$ level.

REFERENCES

1. Åstrand PO, Rodahl K: Textbook of Work Physiology. 3rd Ed. McGraw-Hill, New York, 1986
2. Pardy RL, Hussain SNA, Machlem PT: The ventilatory pump in exercise. Clin Chest Med 5:35, 1984
3. Blackie SP, Fairborn MS, McElvany NG et al: Normal values and ranges for ventilation and breathing pattern at maximal exercise. Chest 100:136, 1991
4. Gowda K, Zintel T, McParland C et al: Diagnostic value of maximal exercise tidal volume. Chest 98:1351, 1990
5. Beachey WD, Olson DE: Quantifying ventilatory reserve to predict respiratory failure in exacerbations of COPD. Chest 97:1087, 1990
6. Bender PR, Martin BJ: Maximal ventilation after exhausting exercise. Med Sci Sports Exerc 17:164, 1985
7. Dempsey JA, Johnson BD, Saupe KW: Adaptations and limitations in the pulmonary system during exercise. Chest suppl 97:S815, 1990
8. Wasserman K, Whipp BJ, Koyal SN, Beaver WL: Anaerobic threshold and respiratory gas exchange during exercise. J Appl Physiol 35:236, 1973
9. Hughes EF, Turner SC, Brooks GA: Effect of glycogen depletion and pedaling speed on anaerobic threshold. J Appl Physiol 52:1598, 1982
10. Farrell SW, Ivy JL: Lactate threshold and the increase in $\dot{V}e/\dot{V}O_2$ during incremental exercise. J Appl Physiol 62:1551, 1987
11. Berry MJ, Stoneman JV, Weyrich AS, Burney B: Dissociation of the ventilatory and lactate thresholds following caffiene ingestion. Med Sci Sports Exer 23:463, 1991
12. Davis HA, Gass GC: The anaerobic threshold as determined before and during lactic acidosis. Eur J Appl Physiol 47:141, 1981
13. Stanley WC, Meess RA, Wisneski JA, Gertz EW: Lactate kinetics during submaxi-

mal exercise in humans: studies with isotopic tracers. J Cardiopulmonary Rehab 9:331, 1988

14. Schneider DA, LaCriox KA, Atkinson GR et al: Ventilatory threshold and maximal oxygen uptake during cycling and running in triathletes. Med Sci Sports Exerc 22:257, 1990
15. Systrom DM, Fragoso CV, Kanarek DJ, Kazemi H: Ammonium ion and the anaerobic threshold in man. Chest 99:1197, 1991
16. Dempsey JA: Is the lung built for exercise? 18:143, 1986
17. Otis AB: The work of breathing. Physiol Rev 34:449, 1954
18. Brice AG, Welch HG: Metabolic and cardiorespiratory responses to He-O$_2$ breathing during exercise. J Appl Physiol: Environ Exer Physiol 54:387, 1983
19. Klinger JR, Hill NS: Right ventricular dysfunction in chronic obstructive pulmonary disease (evaluation and management). Chest 99:715, 1991
20. Morrison DA, Adcock K, Collins CM et al: Right ventricular dysfunction and the exercise limitation of chronic obstructive pulmonary disease. J Am Coll Cardiol 9:1219, 1987
21. Lockhart AT, Nader FL, Schrijen F, Sadoul P: Elevated pulmonary artery wedge pressure at rest and during exercise in chronic bronchitis: fact or fancy? Clin Sci 37:503, 1969
22. Jezek V, Schrizen F, Sadoul P: Right ventricular function and pulmonary hemodynamics during exercise in patients with chronic obstructive pulmonary disease. Cardiology 58:20, 1973
23. Hickam JB, Cargill WH: Effect of exercise on cardiac output and pulmonary arterial pressure in normal persons and in patients with cardiovascular disease and pulmonary emphysema. J Clin Invest 27:10, 1948

3 Exercise Pathophysiology: Pulmonary Impairment

Cynthia Coffin Zadai
Scot Irwin

The efficient and effective response of the pulmonary system to exercise depends on each of the multiple links in the chain from ventilation and external respiration to gas transport and internal respiration. Chapter 2 presents these linkages chronologically, describing the incremental and total potential response to oxygen demand in an individual without pathology. This chapter explores the pulmonary systemic impairments produced by pathologic processes that alter the anticipated pulmonary response to oxygen demand. Becklake et al.[1] have described respiratory impairment as the dysfunction of any or all of the components of the respiratory apparatus (lungs, pleura, chest wall, and muscles, including the diaphragm, and the neurologic control of breathing).

Except for respiratory failure, the pulmonary system is less often considered a culprit in the differential diagnosis of systemic limitation to exercise or response to increased oxygen demand.[2,3] There has been extensive clinical study at both ends of the spectrum between acute and chronic respiratory failure to determine the precipitants and components of failure as well as to evaluate the therapeutic measures used to prevent or resolve failure. These studies have illustrated the range and complexity of the components of the pulmonary system and its capacity to respond to demands for increased oxygen consumption. Under normal conditions and in the absence of pathology, the pulmonary system appears to have a reserve capacity in excess of most oxygen uptake ($\dot{V}O_2$) demands including maximum exercise.[4,5] Less than 10 percent of the vital capacity (VC) is required as tidal volume (Vt) to adequately inflate alveoli, allowing O_2 and CO_2 exchange sufficient to arterialize pulmonary capillary blood at rest.[6] Only two-thirds of the Vt comes into contact with the pulmonary capillary surface area, which accommodates approximately 10 percent of the circulating blood volume[7] to achieve successful gas exchange. The ventilatory muscle contraction rate (or respiratory rate [RR]) at rest is less than 20 percent of rates documented at maximum exercise and only a fraction of the muscles' documented contraction maximum.[5,8] The oxygen consumed by the muscles ($\dot{V}O_2$ resp) to contract at that rate is 2 percent or less of the total body $\dot{V}O_2$ at rest.[5,9,10] Activity demanding maximum oxygen uptake ($\dot{V}O_2$ max) in the nonpathologic subject has not been shown to exceed the pulmonary system's maximum reserves of volume, RR, or gas exchange (Table 3-1).

Increased $\dot{V}O_2$ in any form will require recruitment of some percentage of the system's reserve capacity to meet the demand. This chapter considers disease processes that limit the response capacity of one or more of the pulmonary system's components in the exercise response chain. Disease limitation can reduce the system's total maximum capacity or reduce the efficiency of any one component's response, thereby increasing the energy cost of a particular activity and enhancing the onset of fatigue.

VENTILATORY PUMP

The ventilatory pump is composed of the skeletal muscles of ventilation that are governed by the intrinsic properties of length, tension, and velocity and respond to voluntary and involuntary neurologic stimuli (see Ch. 1). Ventilatory muscle contraction generates a force that displaces the abdominal contents and chest wall (elastic work of breathing), inflating the lung and initiating gas flow (flow resistive work) through the airways.[11] The work performed by the ventilatory pump is referred to as the work of breathing (WOB), and the oxygen consumed by the ventilatory muscles ($\dot{V}O_2$ resp) as the oxygen cost of breathing. The pump's working capacity is measured in terms of total volume of gas that

Table 3-1. Pulmonary System Components and Their Potential Maximum Capacity

Potential Maximum Capacity	Pulmonary System Components				
	Rate	Vt:VC	$\dot{V}O_2$ resp:$\dot{V}O_2$	$\dot{Q}$ pulm capillary:CO	MVV
Rest	10	10%	2%[5,9,10]	10%[7]	5%
Exercise maximum	50	50%	14–20%[5,32]	10%[7]	50–80%[5]
Measured maximum	300–420[8]	100%	?	?	100%

Abbreviations: Vt, tidal volume, VC, vital capacity; $\dot{V}O_2$, maximum oxygen uptake; $\dot{V}O_2$ resp, oxygen consumed by muscles; Q pulm capillary, cardiac output by the pulmonary capillaries; MVV, maximum voluntary ventilation.

can be moved over time in response to $\dot{V}O_2$. The working capacity is expressed and described in measurable terms such as the minute ventilation ($\dot{V}e$ = RR × Vt), which can be recorded at rest or with activity such as maximum exercise ($\dot{V}e:\dot{V}O_2$ max).

Normal subjects exercised to maximum capacity use approximately 50 percent of the VC for $\dot{V}t$ at an RR of 50 to 60 to achieve maximum $\dot{V}e$.[12] The $\dot{V}O_2$ resp for this activity has been calculated at rates of approximately 10 to 20 percent of total body $\dot{V}O_2$[13] (see Ch. 2). These values indicate there is a potential ventilatory pump reserve capacity in the normal individual even at maximum levels of O_2 demand. Pathologic processes that interfere with the ventilatory pump's response to O_2 demand can reduce the efficiency and magnitude of the musculoskeletal response and increase the relative O_2 cost of an activity by increasing either the elastic or flow resistive workload imposed on the ventilatory pump.[5,11]

Impairment

At rest, diaphragmatic contraction is responsible for performing the majority of the WOB by compressing and displacing the abdominal contents, which lifts the lower rib cage up and out.[14] With increasing $\dot{V}O_2$ demand, the intercostals are recruited to assist in lateral and upward chest wall displacement, inflating the rib cage.[15] The total muscle force generated depends on the following factors: a threshold stimulus to initiate contraction, an effective resting muscle length, and an adequate contraction velocity to overcome the load or resistance imposed by the system. Leith and Bradley[16] demonstrated that the ventilatory muscles of normal subjects are skeletal muscles capable of generating effective contractions against progressively greater loads and for increasingly longer amounts of time. Roussos and Macklem[17] showed that at ventilatory loads of less than 40 percent maximum capacity, the ventilatory muscles could continue repetitive contractions for indefinite periods of time. However, conditions (e.g., hypoxia) that either reduced the muscles' capacity to generate force (maximum inspiratory/expiratory pressures [MIP, MEP]) or increased the workload demand above 40 percent maximum capacity produced fatigue and failure in normal subjects, as evidenced by pressure reduction and muscle electromyography (EMG).[17,18] Similarly, clinical studies performed on subjects with pathology that had reduced the skeletal muscles' maximum capacity and/or increased the elastic and flow resistive WOB also elicited signs and symptoms of fatigue and failure in the ventilatory pump.[17-22] Cohen et al.[23] described the fatigue/failure process as observed clinically in patients progressing from EMG fatigue to ventilatory pump failure including (1) increased rate of breathing, (2) discoordinated/asynchronous breathing, (3) paradoxical abdominal/chest wall motion, and (4) increased partial arterial pressure of carbon dioxide ($PaCO_2$).

Diseases and conditions that limit the strength and endurance of ventilatory pump muscles include neurologic conditions that interfere with nerve conduction and muscle contraction, such as polio, myasthenia gravis, Guillain-Barré syndrome, spinal cord trauma, cerebrovascular accident (CVA), Parkinson's disease, amyotrophic lateral sclerosis (ALS), and muscular dystrophy (MD).[22,24,25] These conditions (Table 3-2) can potentially limit the efficiency and magnitude of the pulmonary response to increased $\dot{V}O_2$ or maximum ventilatory capacity ($\dot{V}e$ max). Pump capacity and potential limitation is measured in terms of maximum vital capacity (VC max), maximum voluntary ventilation (MVV), MIP and MEP and maximal sustainable ventilatory capacity (MSVC). Normal values are shown in Table 3-3. Conditions modifying the muscles' ability to respond also include those that affect the muscles' intrinsic properties of length,

Table 3-2. Physiologic Consequences of Pathology That Impairs Ventilatory Pump and Gas Exchange Mechanisms

Pulmonary Impairment	Potential Physiologic Compromise
Neuromuscular Pathology	
Spinal cord compression/transection	
C4–C6	↑ work/accessories; ↓ intrathoracic volume
T1–T12	↑ work/diaphragm and accessories; ↓ intrathoracic volume
Cerebrovascular accident with thoracic involvement	
Paralyzed intercostals	↓ chest wall compliance and volume; ↑ elastic WOB
Paralyzed hemidiaphragm	↓ MIP, MEP, and volume; ↑ elastic WOB
Muscular dystrophy	↓ chest wall compliance
Polio	↑ elastic WOB; ↓ lung volume
Guillain-Barré syndrome	↓ MIP, MEP, and lung compliance
Musculoskeletal Pathology	
Rib fractures	↓ chest wall compliance, lung compliance, and volume; atelectasis; $\dot{V}:\dot{Q}$ mismatch
Kyphoscoliosis	↓ chest wall compliance, lung compliance, and volume; Δ in length/tension/force generation; atelectasis; $\dot{V}:\dot{Q}$ mismatch
Obesity	↑ elastic WOB; ↓ chest wall compliance and lung compliance
Cardiopulmonary Pathology	
Asthma	↓ airway diameter; ↑ flow resistance, airway obstruction, retained volume, and WOB
Atelectasis	↓ lung compliance; ↑ flow resistance and elastic WOB; $\dot{V}:\dot{Q}$ mismatch
Pneumonia	↑ airway obstruction; $\dot{V}:\dot{Q}$ mismatch
Pulmonary edema, CHF	↓ lung compliance and elastic WOB; $\dot{V}:\dot{Q}$ mismatch
COPD	↓ chest wall compliance; ↑ volume retention and airway obstruction; Δ in length/tension/force generation

Abbreviations: ↑, increased; ↓, decreased; Δ, change; WOB, work of breathing; COPD, chronic obstructive pulmonary disease; CHF, congestive heart failure; $\dot{V}$, volume; $\dot{Q}$, cardiac output.

Table 3-3. Normal Values for Ventilatory Pump Functions

Measurements of Ventilatory Pump Function	Normal Values
Volume	
VC	75% of total lung capacity
Vt	10–15% of VC
Flow	
FEV_1	FEV_1:FVC = 80–100%
PEF (predicted)	PEF (L/sec) = 4.63 + 2.385^a − 0.026A^b
Rate	
RR	10–12
Strength	
MIP	Males: 103–124 cm H_2O^{c}
	Females: 65–87 cm H_2O^{c}
MEP	Males: 185–233 cm H_2O^{c}
	Females: 128–152 cm H_2O^{c}
Endurance	
MVV (predicted)	MVV = FEV_1 × 35
MSVC	60% of MVV^d

Abbreviations: Vt, tidal volume; VC, vital capacity; FEV_1, forced expiratory volume in one second; RR, respiratory rate; MIP, maximum inspiratory pressure; MEP, maximum expiratory pressure; MVV, maximum voluntary ventilation; MSVC, maximum sustainable ventilatory capacity; FVC, forced vital capacity; PEF, peak expiratory flow.

^{a} Body surface area in square meters.
^{b} Age in years. (From Bass.[54])
^{c} Mean values ± 2 SD. (From Black and Hyatt.[55])
^{d} From Rochester et al.[37]

tension, and velocity. If the weakened or inefficient muscle is required to contract from a shortened position against a relatively large resistance and the contraction must be rapid as during exercise, the onset of fatigue and failure will occur sooner.

Pathologic processes that increase the WOB can generally be grouped into those that affect the elastic workload and those that increase the flow resistive WOB. Conditions that decrease lung–thorax compliance and/or reduce airway diameter fall into these categories (Table 3-2).[11,22,24,26] Subjects with a rigid thorax and high resistance to abdominal compression and displacement will require greater force of muscle contraction to achieve intrapleural and intrathoracic pressure changes adequate for lung expansion. Similarly, processes that decrease lung volume, collapse alveoli, and increase intra-alveolar surface tension (atelectasis, pneumonia, pulmonary edema) will also demand increased muscle tension to distend and inflate a stiffer lung.[3,6,11] Conversely, pathology that produces air trapping (emphysema, asthma) can decrease elastic recoil and increase residual volume, altering the resting position of the thorax and the breathing pattern and decreasing the expiratory flow rate which increases the elastic WOB.[21,27,28]

Factors that decrease the radius of the airway lumen or retard and prevent its distension during inspiration increase the flow resistive WOB. Airway compression by engorged pulmonary vasculature or overdistended alveoli, airway occlusion with retained secretions, bronchospasm or airway swelling, obstructed airway collapse, and decreased airway elasticity can all contribute to increased flow resistance (Table 3-2).[3,6,11] Physiologic indicators of an increased workload can include (1) a reduced VC despite volume-corrected normal values for MIP and MEP, (2) a reduced inspiratory and/or expiratory flow rate measured by flow–volume loop or spirometry, and (3) increased airway resistance (sGaw) and development of a discoordinated or asynchronous breathing pattern at rest or with activity.[11,21,22,24,25,29]

Response to Exercise

The mechanical ventilatory pump response (force and frequency of muscle contraction) to increased $\dot{V}O_2$ demand is directly proportional to the amount and type of load presented[30] (see Ch. 2). Diseases that cause pulmonary system impairment may require the less impaired links in the exercise response chain to compensate for the weaker links. For example, a muscle functioning in a shortened and mechanically disadvantaged position would potentially be unable to displace the chest wall far enough to create an adequate pressure and volume change for a given $\dot{V}e$ and $\dot{V}O_2$ demand. However, by increasing RR, the rate component could potentially compensate for the impaired volume response and still achieve an adequate $\dot{V}e$ to meet the $\dot{V}O_2$ demand of exercise.

Although the $\dot{V}O_2$ goal may be attained under the previously described conditions, a careful look at the O_2 cost under such conditions is required. The ventilatory pump work involved requires a larger number of muscle contractions to achieve $\dot{V}O_2$. A higher RR increases the $\dot{V}O_2$ resp above that normally required and decreases the proportion of $\dot{V}O_2$ available to other exercising muscles.[22,26,31] The contractions performed at a higher velocity also generate potentially less force per contraction at a greater O_2 cost, decreasing the efficiency of the ventilatory pump.[5,14,17,26] Aerobic properties of the ventilatory muscles (high capillary density, high percentage aerobic enzymes) ensure a high rate of O_2 delivery during any activity, potentially at the expense of other skeletal muscles.[13,32,33]

The physiology of the ventilatory pump response to exercise in chronic obstructive pulmonary disease (COPD) provides a good illustration of the complex interactions when a pathologically impaired pump responds to an increased O_2 demand or when the ventilatory workload associated with pump response exceeds the system's maximum supply capacity. Figure 3-1 depicts the resting anatomic position of the ventilatory pump in COPD and a flow volume loop of a normal individual compared to that of an individual with COPD.[22,24,34] The volume retention associated with COPD has decreased elastic recoil pressure and expiratory flow[35] while changing the resting position of the thorax (partial inspiration at end expiration) to include a more horizontal position of the lower rib pairs, lower resting position of the diaphragm, and shortening of the diaphragm's resting length. The altered angle of pull during diaphragmatic contraction decreases the efficiency of pump mechanics by reducing the amount of

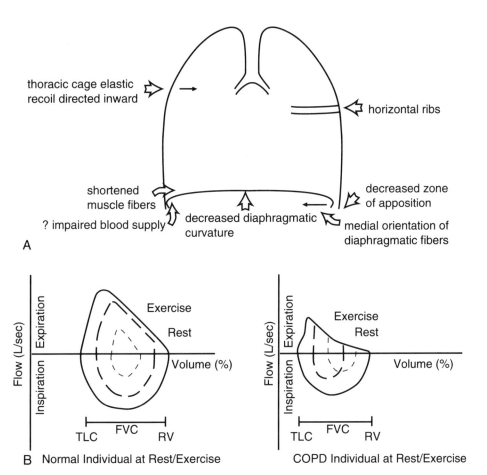

Fig. 3-1. **(A)** Physiologic effects of altered chest wall position in chronic obstructive pulmonary disease (COPD) with hyperinflation. (From Tobin,[22] with permission.) **(B)** Flow–volume loops at rest and with activity. (From Zadai,[34] with permission.)

caudad and lateral abdominal displacement, with the resultant rib cage lift decreasing the amount of intrapleural and intrathoracic pressure change for a given muscle tension.[22,14,24] Muscle force potential has also decreased due to its shortened length.

The flow–volume loop of the normal individual illustrates the reserve capacity available for the increased demands of exercise. Faster, more forceful muscle contraction during inspiration increases inspiratory flow and volume and essentially primes the pump to take advantage of the steep expiratory flow curve during active expiration and most efficiently accomplish the WOB.[5,34,36] The flow–volume loop in COPD (Fig. 3-1) indicates that when the subject is breathing at $\dot{V}t$, he is already taking advantage of his maximum expiratory flow rate to exhale at rest.[36] Any attempt the COPD patient makes to increase respiratory rate, volume, and flow will compound the mechanical length tension–velocity disadvantage predisposing the muscles to fatigue and the system to mechanical failure.[28,36–38]

The $\dot{V}O_2$ resp associated with resting Vt for such a mechanically disadvantaged and inefficient pump is similar to that calculated for normal individuals during low level ambulation.[31] To increase ventilation and meet the $\dot{V}O_2$ demand of activity, this subject would have to increase his Vt and RR. The physiologic consequences of meeting that $\dot{V}O_2$ demand would include the following:

1. Increasing intrathoracic volume further reduces muscle length, decreasing the muscle's remaining mechanical advantage.
2. The increased velocity of muscle contraction decreases force generation potential.
3. The greater muscle contraction force required to increase flow rate during expiration can actually compress airways, increasing flow resistance and trapping further volume.
4. Increased air trapping decreases rather than increases the efficiency of gas exchange.

Several studies have investigated the ability to maintain increased minute ventilation as an indicator of endurance capacity in subjects with COPD (Fig. 3-2). Because the $\dot{V}e$ requirement is such a high percentage of MVV, fatigue and failure occur earlier.[39–42]

Studies examining the oxygen cost of breathing for COPD subjects at rest have calculated $\dot{V}O_2$ resp in the 30 ml/min range, or approximately 15 percent of the body's total resting $\dot{V}O_2$.[9,31,43] $\dot{V}O_2$ resp increases curvilinearly with increasing $\dot{V}O_2$ demands and higher levels of $\dot{V}e$ (Fig. 3-3).[5,31,32] Increased $\dot{V}O_2$ demands in such individuals require increased $\dot{V}e$ at an exorbitant $\dot{V}O_2$ resp cost. Because the MVV is also dramatically reduced, $\dot{V}e$ max is rapidly reached. The increased $\dot{V}O_2$ demand of low level ambulation in severely compromised COPD patients could therefore easily exceed their $\dot{V}O_2$ max in minutes, with most of the increase in $\dot{V}O_2$ being consumed by the ventilatory muscles.[9,13,31,32,43]

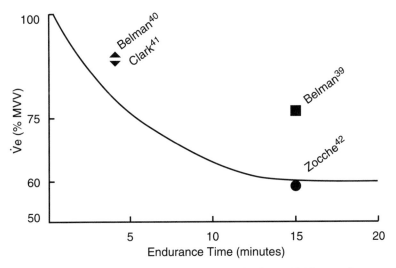

Fig. 3-2. Relationship of maximum voluntary ventilation (MVV) to endurance time in subjects with chronic obstructive pulmonary disease (COPD). The relationship between endurance time and minute ventilation is expressed as a percentage of MVV. Healthy subjects can sustain approximately 60 percent of MVV indefinitely (maximal sustainable ventilatory capacity [MSVC]). Data obtained in four studies of patients with COPD are shown. (From Tobin,[22] with permission, as adapted from Rochester DF, Arora NS, Braun NMT et al: The respiratory muscles in chronic obstructive pulmonary disease [COPD] Bull Europ Physiopath Resp 15:951, 1979.)

PULMONARY GAS EXCHANGE

The primary goal of ventilatory pump activity is to provide an adequate volume of air for gas exchange. At rest, the Vt required to accomplish this exchange is approximately 10 percent of the VC.[6] Approximately two-thirds of each Vt breath reaches the alveolar level to participate in gas exchange (alveolar ventilation [$\dot{V}_A$]). The remaining third of the Vt is accommodated in the anatomic dead space (V_D) and exits at the beginning of expiration (Vt = V_D + $\dot{V}_A$). The V_D is comprised of the trachea, mainstem bronchi, and conducting airways, which change only slightly with exercise as they distend to accommodate a larger gas volume. The alveoli, however, have the capacity to open and distend, accommodating progressively larger volumes of gas with increasing O_2 demand. The amount of gas reaching the alveoli to participate in gas exchange is dependent both on the ventilatory pump factors previously described and on the breathing pattern chosen to deliver the minute ventilation ($\dot{V}e$ = RR × Vt). A 6 ft, 70 kg male with a Vt of 500 ml will have a V_D of approximately 150 ml, or

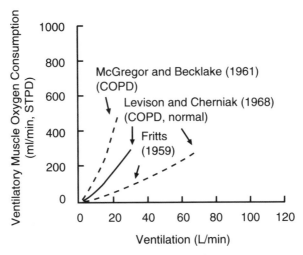

Fig. 3-3. Ventilatory muscle oxygen consumption ($\dot{V}O_2$ resp) in relation to ventilation ($\dot{V}e$) during exercise and voluntary hyperpnea in normal subjects, and in exercise and hyperventilation in patients with chronic obstructive pulmonary disease. (COPD). (Adapted from Pardy et al.,[5] with permission.)

one-third the Vt. At a resting (minute ventilation) $\dot{V}e$ of 5 L/min, one-third of the $\dot{V}e$ (1.5 L/min) would have ventilated the dead space rather than participating in $\dot{V}_A$:

$$[\dot{V}e = (RR \times \dot{V}t)], \text{ or } [5 \text{ L/min} = (10 \times 500 \text{ ml/min})] =$$
$$10 \,(350 \text{ ml/min} + 150\text{ml/min})$$

An increased $\dot{V}O_2$ demand that doubled the $\dot{V}e$ requirement of this individual would be most efficiently achieved by maintaining the same RR and maximally increasing Vt.[5,6] Because the V_D remains essentially the same, the majority of the volume increase would be accommodated at the alveolar level:

$$\dot{V}e \,(10 \text{ L/min}) = 10 \,(850 \text{ ml/min} + 150 \text{ ml/min})$$

Inability to effectively increase Vt puts the ventilatory pump at a disadvantage for efficient gas exchange. The same individual described earlier with a minute ventilation requirement of 10 L/min who is forced to rely on RR to meet the demand could have the following result:

$$\dot{V}e \,(10 \text{ L/min}) = 20 \,(350 \text{ mL/min} + 150 \text{ mL/min})$$

At an RR of ten, the total V_D is 1.5 L/min, whereas at a rate of 20, the V_D is doubled (3.0 L/min), with a resultant decline in $\dot{V}_A$. Pulmonary pathology that impairs chest wall motion (e.g., muscle fatigue and failure) or alveolar distention (e.g., pulmonary edema) can thereby reduce efficiency of gas exchange (Table 3-2).

Once a given volume of air has reached the alveolar level, gas exchange is dependent on the partial pressure of alveolar gases, available surface area, diffusion time and distance, and pulmonary circulation.[6] The partial pressures and molecular weights of O_2 and CO_2 at sea level create the physiologic advantage that drives oxygen from the alveolus into the pulmonary capillary and carbon dioxide from venous blood into the alveolus (see Fig. 2-6). Effective maintenance of the alveolar (P_AO_2) to arterial (PaO_2) partial pressure of oxygen during exercise depends on rapid gas exchange over a large surface area. Actual alveolar surface area has been calculated at approximately 80 m^2 for the 70 kg, 6 ft male mentioned earlier and the pulmonary circulation covers 80 to 95 percent of the alveolar surface, providing a potential gas exchange surface area of 70 m^2.[44,45] Recruitment of this surface area in response to O_2 demand occurs progressively with increasing levels of alveolar distention. Simultaneously, pulmonary vascular changes must occur to allow for an increase in the volume and speed of circulation blood.[46] The matching of ventilation to circulation is described as the ratio of alveolar ventilation to cardiac output ($\dot{Q}$), or $\dot{V}_A:\dot{Q}$.

Accommodations of the circulatory system to exercise include changes in pressure and flow (Table 3-4).[6,46] The collective increase in $\dot{Q}$ and pulmonary arterial pressures while the vasculature dilates and resistance falls allows for an increased volume of blood to be evenly distributed and quickly transported through the lung. The total result of increased $\dot{V}e$ and circulation is improved throughout $\dot{V}_A:\dot{Q}$ the lung and rapid, effective gas exchange.

Table 3-4. Comparison of Pulmonary and Systemic Hemodynamic Variables During Rest and Exercise of Moderate Severity in the Normal Adult Male

Condition	Rest (Sitting)	Exercise
Oxygen consumption	300	2,000 ml/min
Blood flow		
Cardiac output	6.3	16.2 L/min
Heart rate	70	135 beats/min
Stroke volume	90	120 ml/beat
Intravascular pressures		
Pulmonary arterial pressure	20/10	30/11 mmHg
Mean	14	20 mmHg
Left atrial pressure, mean	8	10 mmHg
Brachial arterial pressure	120/70	155/78 mmHg
Mean	88	112 mmHg
Right atrial pressure, mean	8	1 mmHg
Resistances		
Pulmonary vascular resistance	0.95	0.62 units[a]
Systemic vascular resistance	13.2	6.9 units[a]

[a] Units = mmHg/L/min.
From Murray,[6] with permission.

Gas Exchange Impairment

Lung pathology has the potential to impair of each component of the gas exchange system. Acute lung disease, such as atelectasis, pneumonia, and pulmonary edema, can fill the alveolar spaces with exudate and fluid or increase intra-alveolar surface tension, preventing distension and producing alveolar collapse.[3,47] COPD fills conducting airways with secretions, destroys the airway support structure, and enlarges terminal airways and alveoli, breaking down alveolar walls. Each process, acute or chronic, increases resistance to airflow and decreases effective $\dot{V}_A$, reducing the $\dot{V}_A:\dot{Q}$ ratio and impairing the efficiency of gas exchange. Pathologic processes that fill or collapse alveoli produce right-to-left shunt, as venous blood will perfuse pulmonary capillaries without receiving O_2, effectively reducing PaO_2. Similarly, pathologic processes that eliminate surface area or decrease the efficacy of $\dot{Q}$ (e.g., left-sided heart failure, COPD) produce an increased amount of V_D, or over-ventilation, without circulation, which also impairs gas exchange.

Reduction and obstruction of either the alveolar or pulmonary capillary surface area initially decreases the available pulmonary reserve capacity to meet the gas exchange requirement of increased O_2 demand. Progressive destruction and reduction over time may eventually impair gas exchange even at rest.[5,26] Similarly, any increased sGaw or increased resistance to blood flow will increase the oxygen cost of oxygen delivery and potentially reduce the oxygen supply available to the system.[32,38,43,48] Physiologic responses at rest or during exercise under conditions of limited gas exchange will demonstrate greater than normal values for a given level of activity and reduced maximum capacity, and may be accompanied by hypoxia, hypercapnia, and early onset of fatigue.[5,24,26]

Response to Exercise

Limitation of exercise due to impaired gas exchange results from lack of O_2 in the arterial blood supplying the exercising muscle and produces an elevation in cellular, venous, and arterial levels of CO_2.[5,24,26,46] Although there are other factors that can contribute to circulatory hypoxia and hypercarbia in addition to the pulmonary pathologies described, the cellular and pulmonary response is similar. The most efficient cellular mechanism for energy liberation is the aerobic production of ATP, consuming O_2 and producing CO_2 (see Ch. 2). The aerobic metabolic breakdown of carbohydrate, protein, or fat depends on a steady delivery of O_2 to the cell and removal of CO_2 from the cell. Any limitation of the O_2 supply will force earlier and more significant use of anaerobic pathways to liberate energy.

All systemic increases in O_2 demand will be met with an increase in O_2 supply, using the gas exchange reserve capacity up to the system's maximum uptake and transport capacity.[6,46] Any limitation of the gas exchange capacity will result in a decreased $\dot{V}O_2$ max and force earlier reliance on a greater percentage of anaerobic metabolism to release energy. This is a rapid and self-limiting mechanism in gas exchange impairment. An increased reliance on anaerobic metabolism increases lactic acid production, lowering cellular and circulatory pH, which impairs cellular metabolism and further stimulates ventilation demand in a disabled system.[5,26,46]

Jones et al.[49] studied pulmonary gas exchange during exercise in COPD patients and found differences in the physiologic responses between study subjects based on individual primary diagnoses. Severe emphysema patients demonstrated a mean decline of 22 mmHg in the PaO_2 during exercise, while chronic bronchitic patients had a mean PaO_2 increase of 6 mmHg (Fig. 3-4). Additionally, the emphysematous patients had a lower workload and higher V_D:Vt ratio than the chronic bronchitics. The authors postulated this difference was due to an improved $\dot{V}_A$:$\dot{Q}$ ratio in the chronic bronchitics as they recruited and opened collapsed alveoli during exercise, while the emphysematous patients had significant alveolar–capillary dysfunction, giving them a fixed $\dot{V}_A$:$\dot{Q}$ ratio. Minh et al.[50] studied 17 COPD patients at maximum exercise and found that those subjects who desaturated had higher functional residual capacities,

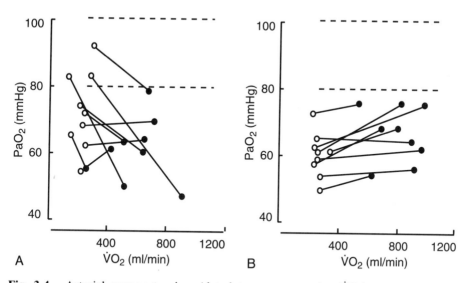

Fig. 3-4. Arterial oxygen tension related to oxygen uptake ($\dot{V}O_2$) at rest and with exercise in **(A)** emphysematous and **(B)** chronic bronchitic patients. The open circles (o) are the resting values, and closed circles (●) are values during exercise. The dotted lines represent the range of partial arterial pressure of oxygen (PaO_2) in normal subjects. Note that six out of nine emphysematous subjects show a drop in PaO_2, but only one out of nine of the chronic bronchitics shows a reduction in PaO_2 with exercise. (From Jones NL et al.,[49] with permission.)

residual volumes, and total lung capacities in combination with lower forced expiratory volume in one second (FEV_1) and maximum breathing capacity than subjects who did not desaturate. Patients who desaturated also demonstrated a significant difference in alveolar to arterial oxygen tension difference $[(A - a) DO_2]$ with a mean decline in PaO_2 from 63 to 53 mmHg and an O_2 saturation (SaO_2) from 91 to 85 percent during exercise. Those subjects who desaturated appeared to have both a high O_2 cost of breathing and an impaired gas exchange capacity.

Arterial desaturation has also been shown to correlate with reductions in diffusing capacity and resting pulmonary hypertension.[26] Raffstein et al.[51] studied 20 COPD patients during exercise whose primary diagnosis was chronic bronchitis. These investigators could group their subjects following the study based on specific arterial blood gas changes that occurred during exercise. Group I patients ($N = 8$) demonstrated a mean decrease in PaO_2 of 7 mmHg, while $PaCO_2$ increased by a mean of 6.5 mmHg. In contrast, group II patients ($N = 12$) had a 2 to 24 mmHg increase in PaO_2 while $PaCO_2$ did not change. A summary comparison of other physiologic data indicated group I had a lower FEV_1 and $FEV_1:FVC$, combined with a lower PaO_2 and higher $PaCO_2$ at rest, than group II. Additionally, group I's pulmonary artery pressure increased from 30 to 54 mmHg during exercise, while group II's range was 24 to 39 mmHg. The authors noted that a larger degree of airway obstruction, hypoxia, and hypercarbia may be associated with a significant degree of pulmonary hypertension and more severe limitation in exercise performance.

Alterations in gas exchange are also associated with acid-base changes during exercise. In a study of patients with chronic airflow obstruction, analysis of blood gases showed increases in $PaCO_2$ and decreases in pH, suggestive of respiratory acidosis.[52] It is well known that during anaerobic metabolism, muscle and blood levels of lactate increase, placing further demands on the respiratory gas exchange mechanism to eliminate CO_2.[46,53] Patients who are unable to meet this demand at rest will be further compromised by exercise.

SUMMARY

Limitation to maximum exercise performance is easily produced by pathologic processes compromising either of the systems responsible for ventilation or respiration. Observation and measurement of pulmonary mechanics and gas exchange at rest and during exercise can assist with documenting the impaired components of the pulmonary system. Diseases that impair neuromuscular contraction of the ventilatory muscles can decrease the strength and endurance of muscle contraction, exposing the muscle to early onset of fatigue and failure in response to increased O_2 demand. Diseases that decrease lung–thorax compliance and increase sGaw increase both WOB and the O_2 cost of ventilatory muscle work. Pathologic changes that decrease $\dot{V}_A$ and pulmonary circulation reduce the gas exchange potential and can decrease the O_2 supply and lessen the ability to eliminate CO_2. Any one of or combination of these factors has the potential to decrease $\dot{V}O_2$ max and increase the relative $\dot{V}O_2$ cost of an activity by decreasing the efficiency of the pulmonary system's response. Physiologic evidence of an impaired pulmonary system limiting exercise response includes (1) an increased $\dot{V}e:\dot{V}O_2$ ratio for a given workload, (2) inability to achieve a ventilatory steady state, (3) low work rate tolerance with rapid progression to maximum capacity, (4) early onset of ventilatory muscle fatigue (asynchronous and discoordinated breathing pattern), and (5) a fall in SaO_2 with a rise in CO_2.

REFERENCES

1. Becklake MR, Rodarte J, Kalica A: National Heart, Lung, and Blood Institute workshop: scientific issues in the assessment of respiratory impairment. Am Rev Respir Dis 137:1505, 1988
2. Snell PG, Mitchell TH: The role of maximal oxygen uptake in exercise performance. Clin Chest Med 5:51, 1984
3. Hedley-Whyte J, Burgess G, Feeley T, Miller M: Applied Physiology of Respiratory Care. Little, Brown, Boston, 1976
4. Bye PT, Farkas GA, Roussos CH: Respiratory factors limiting exercise. Annu Rev Physiol 45:439, 1983
5. Pardy RL, Hussain SNA, Macklem PT: The ventilatory pump in exercise. Clin Chest Med 5:35, 1984
6. Murray JF: The Normal Lung. WB Saunders, Philadelphia, 1976
7. DeFreitas FM, Faraco EZ, Deazevedo DF et al: Behavior of normal pulmonary circulation during changes of total blood volume in man. J Clin Invest 44:366, 1965
8. Otis AB, Guyatt AR: The maximal frequency of breathing of man at various tidal volumes. Respir Physiol 5:118, 1968
9. Campbell EJM: Westlake EK, Cherniak RM: Simple methods of estimating oxygen consumption and efficiency of the muscles of breathing. J Appl Physiol 11:303, 1957
10. Milic-Emili G, Petit JM, Deroanne R: Mechanical work of breathing during exercise in trained and untrained subjects. J Appl Physiol 17:43, 1962
11. Derenne JPH, Macklem PT, Roussos CH: The respiratory muscles: mechanics, control and pathophysiology (parts I, II, III). Am Rev Respir Dis 118:119, 1978
12. Jensen JI, Lyager S, Pedersen OF: The relationship between maximal ventilation, breathing pattern and mechanical limitation of ventilation. J Physiol 309:521, 1980
13. Roussos CH, Macklem PT: The respiratory muscles. N Engl J Med 307:786, 1982
14. Luce JM, Culver BH: Respiratory muscle function in health and disease. Chest 81:82, 1982
15. Taylor A: Contribution of the intercostal muscles to the effort of respiration in man. J Physiol 151:390, 1960
16. Leith D, Bradley M: Ventilatory muscle strength and endurance training. J Appl Physiol 41:508, 1976
17. Roussos CH, Macklem PT: Diaphragmatic fatigue in man. J Appl Physiol 43:897, 1977
18. Macklem PT: Respiratory muscles: The vital pump. Chest 78:753, 1980
19. Byrd RB, Hyatt RE: Maximal respiratory pressures in chronic obstructive lung disease. Am Rev Respir Dis 98:848, 1968

20. Braun NMT, Rochester DF: Respiratory muscle function in obstructive pulmonary disease. Am Rev Respir Dis 115:91, 1977
21. Ashutosh K, Gilbert R, Auchincloss J et al: Asynchronous breathing movements in patients with chronic obstructive pulmonary disease. Chest 67:553, 1975
22. Tobin MJ: Respiratory muscles in disease. Clin Chest Med 9:264, 1988
23. Cohen CA, Zagelbaum G, Gross D et al: Clinical manifestations of inspiratory muscle fatigue. Am J Med 73:308, 1982
24. Aldrich TK: Respiratory muscle fatigue. Clin Chest Med 9:225, 1988
25. Aldrich TK, Aldrich MS: Primary muscle diseases. In Kamholz SL (ed): Pulmonary Aspects of Neurologic Diseases. PMA Publishing, New York, 1987
26. Loke J, Mahler DA, Paul-Man SF et al: Exercise impairment in chronic obstructive pulmonary disease. Clin Chest Med 5:121, 1984
27. Potter WA, Olafsson S, Hyatt RE: Ventilatory mechanics and expiratory flow limitation during exercise in patients with obstructive lung disease. J Clin Invest 50:910, 1971
28. Grimby G, Elgefors B, Oxhøj H: Ventilatory levels and chest wall mechanics during exercise in obstructive lung disease. Scand J Clin Lab Invest 25:303, 1970
29. Aldrich TK, Arora NS, Rochester DF: The influence of airway obstruction and ventilatory muscle strength on maximum voluntary ventilation in lung disease. Am Rev Respir Dis 126:195, 1982
30. Jensen JI, Lyager S, Pederson OF: The relationship between maximal ventilation, breathing pattern and mechanical limitation of ventilation. J Physiol 309:521, 1980
31. Levison H, Cherniack RM: Ventilatory cost of exercise in chronic obstructive pulmonary disease. J Appl Physiol 25:21, 1968
32. McGregor M, Becklake MR: The relationship of oxygen cost of breathing to respiratory mechanical work and respiratory force. J Clin Invest 40:971, 1961
33. Shephard RJ: The oxygen cost of breathing during vigorous exercise. Q J Exp Physiol 51:336, 1966
34. Zadai CC: Therapeutic exercise in pulmonary disease and disability. p. 412 In: Basmajian JV, Wolf SL (eds): Therapeutic Exercise. 5th Ed. Williams & Wilkins, Baltimore, 1990
35. Gibson GT, Pride NB: Lung distensibility: the static pressure–volume curve of the lungs and its use in clinical assessment. Br J Dis Chest 70:143, 1976
36. Leaver DJ, Pride NB: Flow volume curves and expiratory pressures during exercise in patients with chronic airway obstruction. Scand J Respir Dis, suppl. 77:S23, 1971
37. Rochester DF, Arora NS, Braun NMT et al: The respiratory muscles in chronic obstructive pulmonary disease. Bull Eur Physiopathol Respir 15:951, 1979
38. Stubbing DJ, Pengelly LD, Morse JLC et al: Pulmonary mechanics during exercise in patients with chronic air flow obstruction. J Appl Physiol 49:506, 1980
39. Belman MJ, Mittman C: Ventilatory muscle training improves exercise capacity in COPD patients. Am Rev Respir Dis 121:273, 1980
40. Belman MJ, Sieck GC, Mozar A: Aminophylline and its influence on ventilatory endurance in humans. Am Rev Respir Dis 131:226, 1985
41. Clark TJH, Freedman S, Campbell EJM et al: The ventilatory capacity of patients with chronic airways obstruction. Clin Sci 36:307, 1969
42. Zocche GP, Fritts HW, Cournand A: Fraction of maximum breathing capacity available for prolonged hyperventilation. J Appl Physiol 15:1073, 1960
43. Cherniack RM: The oxygen consumption and efficiency of respiratory muscles in health and emphysema. J Clin Invest 38:494, 1959
44. Weibel ER: Morphometry of the Human Lung. Springer-Verlag, Berlin, 1961

45. Weibel ER: Morphological basis of alveolar–capillary gas exchange. Physiol Rev 53:419, 1973

46. Åstrand PO, Rodahl K: Textbook of Work Physiology. 3rd Ed. McGraw Hill, New York, 1986

47. Robbins S, Cotran R, Kumar V: Pathologic Basis of Disease. WB Saunders, Philadelphia, 1984

48. Belman MJ, Wasserman K: Exercise training and testing in patients with chronic obstruction disease. Basics Resp Dis 10:1, 1981

49. Jones NL et al: Pulmonary gas exchange during exercise in patients with chronic airway obstruction. Clin Sci 31:39, 1966

50. Minh VD, Lee HM, Dolan GF et al: Hypoxemia during exercise in patients with chronic obstructive pulmonary disease. Am Rev Respir Dis 120:787, 1979

51. Raffstein B, Escourrou P, LeGrand A et al: Circulatory transport of oxygen in patients with chronic airflow obstruction exercising maximally. Am Rev Respir Dis 125:426, 1982

52. Nery LE, Wasserman K, French W et al: Contrasting cardiovascular and respiratory responses to exercise in mitral value and chronic obstructive pulmonary disease. Chest 83:446, 1983

53. Wasserman K, Whipp BJ: Exercise physiology in health and disease. Am Rev Respir Dis 112:219, 1975

54. Bass H: The flow volume loop: normal standards and abnormalities in chronic obstructive pulmonary disease. Chest 63:171, 1973

55. Black LF, Hyatt RE: Maximal respiratory pressures: normal values and relationship to age and sex. Am Rev Respir Dis 69:696, 1969

4

Comprehensive Physical Therapy Evaluation: Identifying Potential Pulmonary Limitations

Cynthia Coffin Zadai

Assessment of the pulmonary system begins the moment the patient is to be examined. Observation and mental notation of the patient's posture; use of musculature; and rate, rhythm, and pattern of breathing occurs whether the subject is walking into the office, sitting in a chair, or sleeping in a bed. The individual's unconscious choices for ventilation (rate, rhythm, pattern) may dramatically change once the active assessment starts, which provides additional information about the patient's pulmonary system. Because the pulmonary system is capable of responding to conscious, subconscious, and physiologic stimuli on a breath-to-breath basis, objective and subjective input and measured responses are all documented.

Examination and assessment can occur in several settings and under a variety of conditions. Observation of ventilation at rest, during activity, and during sleep can all contribute to the diagnosis of acute and chronic ventilatory and respiratory impairments (impairment deficits) and measure response to a variety of changing conditions. The World Health Organization (WHO) defines health in terms of complete physical, mental, and social well-being.[1] Investigators have attempted to further classify health in terms of physical, mental, emotional, and social function.[2] The physical therapist primarily examines the patient to identify impairments (anatomic or physiologic abnormality or loss of an organ or system)[2,3] that limit physical function and can be altered by treatment.[4] This chapter presents a method approach to observation, assessment, and interpretation of pulmonary signs, symptoms, and tests of ventilation and gas exchange to identify impairments that limit physical function.

THORACIC PHYSICAL EXAMINATION

Observation and Interview

The initial step in examining a patient includes an interview and observation of the ventilatory pump at rest. Reasonable exposure of the thorax during the interview allows the observer to note musculoskeletal abnormalities, pattern of breathing, and specific ventilatory muscle use. The interview includes questions regarding past medical and surgical history, history of the present illness, the individual's present functional level (activities of daily living [ADL] and work history), social history, and the patient's subjective complaints (see Table 4-1). Patients who do not historically have pulmonary diagnoses may have indicators of pulmonary dysfunction when describing symptoms elicited during performance of activities such as walking, driving, or lying in their most comfortable sleeping position (use of three pillows).

Past medical and surgical history, such as frequent upper respiratory infections or seasonal exacerbations of dyspnea requiring medication, can establish a pattern for pulmonary disease. Symptoms such as night or morning cough and progressive dyspnea with minimal activity will also alert the examiner to possibilities of pulmonary pathology. Careful interviewing can elicit the objective signs and symptoms and the patient's personal response to or feeling about the symptoms. "Do you do your own grocery shopping?" may reveal useful information in a variety of areas. Is the patient independent in ADL? Is there an intact support system? Can the patient walk, climb stairs, drive to and from the store or carry packages, etc.? Are there symptoms elicited during specific segments of daily activity? Does the patient perceive himself or herself as dependant or self-sustaining? How does the patient respond to that perception? Each response during the interview can be an indicator of how self-aware the subject is, how much education the subject will require regarding the disease process, how well motivated the individual will be for self-care or return to work, and upon what realistic goals the therapist and individual would be able to agree.

Objective observations during patient interview range from skin color and facial expression to the actual respiratory rate (RR) and pattern of chest wall motion during resting ventilation. Is the motion bilaterally symmetrical and synchronous, and are accessory muscles used? Mental notes on the patient's initial presentation establish a baseline against which changes in the patient can be judged during subjection to a range of conditions occurring in the interview and assessment. Respiratory rate at rest or with activity can be an indicator of

Table 4-1. Patient Interview

Type of Interview Questions	Details Covered
General	Past medical history, allergies, medication use Past surgical history, hospitalizations Family medical history: parents, siblings, children
Specific	History of present illness to include onset of signs and symptoms (date, time, frequency) of cough, temperature, congestion, chills, and/or sweats, dyspnea, pain, dizziness, nausea
Functional activity history	Work history, ambulatory ability, walking distance or taking stairs, independence in activities of daily living, exercise history, environmental effects (season, temperature, etc.), sleeping pattern
Social history	Support system/family, past/present social habits (ETOH, smoking), past/present living location, avocations

oxygen demand and ventilatory pump work. The pattern of ventilation may indicate the presence of neurologic disease (Cheyne-Stokes ventilation), metabolic disease (Kussmaul breathing), musculoskeletal impairment (flail chest and paradoxic motion) or obstructive pulmonary disease (pursed lip exhalation). Position and use of musculature may indicate clinical conditions such as impending respiratory failure (RR 50 breaths per minute and an inability to breathe other than when sitting upright, supported by the upper extremities and using all accessory muscles).

Normal values and patterns are described in Table 4-2 to illustrate the range

Table 4-2. Physical Examination and Observation: Normal Values and Patterns

Physical Aspect	Signs and Symptoms
Posture	Standing/sitting/supine position Active muscle contraction: diaphragm, intercostals, abdominal, accessories Symetrical chest wall: clavicle/scapula position, appropriate vertebral curves, sternal position
Thoracic/abdominal motion	Respiratory rate: infant, (40–50 breaths per minute at rest, 120 with activity); adult, (10–12 breaths per minute at rest, 50 with activity) Rhythm: inspiratory-to-expiratory ratio 1 : 2 at rest, 1 : 1 with activity Tidal breaths note: slight increase in anteroposterior diameter, symetrical increase in lateral basal diameter, increased abdominal excursion at end inspiration No supraclavicular, subcostal or intercostal retraction; no asymetric or paradoxical chest wall/abdominal motion; no pursed lip breathing, stridor, or grunting
Appearance	Skin: normal flesh tone versus ruddy, cyanotic, or jaundiced; cool, clammy, dry Awake, alert, responsive
Head and neck	Facial expression, nasal flaring versus mouth breathing Mouth: assess for tongue control, dentures, swallowing, midline trachea, effective cough

of signs and symptoms that interview questions should cover to provide a basis for evaluating change. Observation is not completed with the first phase of examination. It continues throughout the complete examination as the value of the observations made initially increases when compared to values noted with each change of position, performance of activity, or change in condition. Alteration from baseline values during progression from rest to performance of ADL, through ambulation, and up to maximum exercise will provide the basis for determining each individual's pulmonary reserve and maximum physical functional capacity.

Palpation, Percussion, and Auscultation

The three components of physical examination that begin to confirm or rule out initial observations as significant are learned skills that become more useful and reliable as they are practiced over time. Palpation and percussion require the assessor to lay hands on the patient and make subjective decisions about chest wall motion, efficacy of muscle contraction, and density of unseen intrathoracic structures. Auscultation employs the most commonly used instrument of measurement in medicine[5]—the stethoscope—and requires a skilled listener to correctly hear and label sounds and to reliably describe the findings in the patient's record or to others who also treat the patient. Although each of these skills has been shown to have variable reliability as an objective clinical measure, they have been shown to be extremely useful as clinical indicators when used among a population of professionals trained in the use of common terms and techniques.[6,7]

Palpation

Palpation of the chest wall can pinpoint areas of localized pain or tenderness, crepitus, and swelling. Muscle contraction and chest wall motion during inspiration and expiration or change in chest wall or abdominal motion during position change can be detected or confirmed with palpation. Chest pain described as "angina" by the patient can be ruled out as such if elicited by the therapist with palpation when the subject is at rest. Diaphragmatic contraction that cannot be observed when the patient is sitting may be palpated in supine when the diaphragm is stretched and facilitated. Increase or decrease in subcostal angle (less than 90 or greater than 110 degrees) observed at rest and confirmed with palpation may indicate the presence of obstructive or restrictive pulmonary disease. However, the range of values documented in a normal population indicates that resting subcostal angle alone is not a reliable indicator of disease presence.[8] Palpation of thoracic excursion is probably best used to assess presence or absence of chest wall motion and symmetry of movement or presence of pain.

Percussion

Percussion is used to discriminate between solid or fluid- and air-filled space intrathoracically. Consequently, percussion findings can be an adjunct to assessing for pneumothorax, diaphragmatic excursion, and presence of plural effusion. Normal resonant percussion note elicited in the first to eleventh intercostal space indicates air filled-lung tissue and should be similar (right) to (left) in each subject. An abnormal percussion note (hyperresonant, dull, or flat) unilaterally or bilaterally may indicate the need for referral to a physician and additional objective testing such as chest x-ray. Comparing change in percussion sound from apex to base and right to left using the subject as the control is most useful to establish a baseline and document change.

Auscultation

Auscultation has been a valuable and essential component of the patient's examination procedure to (1) immediately detect acute change such as degree of airway patency or congestive failure; (2) document response to bronchopulmonary hygiene, bronchodilators, and controlled breathing patterns; or (3) rule out or document a positive response to treatment over time. The value of auscultation as a clinical assessment tool was first described in 1761 by Auenbrugger,[9] who discussed its possible advantages and limitations. These advantages and limitations have been studied and described many times in the more than two centuries that have passed.[10,11] Achieving consensus on terminology has been the most useful step toward increasing the reliability of this clinical assessment tool[12] (see Table 4-3).

Use of the stethoscope to auscultate breath sounds and voice sounds at rest and with activity provides information across a range of conditions. Classification of "normal" auscultated sound into bronchial or tracheal sounds heard over the airways and vesicular sounds heard over lung tissue simplifies reporting. Any variation from baseline such as decreased or absent breath sounds is characterized as abnormal. Progression of lung collapse or fluid accumulation during activity or change in position can be detected simply with monitoring over time. Additional sounds are categorized as adventitious and further divided into continuous or discontinuous sounds. These are commonly heard when secretions or interstitial fluid accumulates in airways or airways are narrowed by swelling or smooth muscle contraction. Voice sounds are reported as decreased, increased or changed in quality (E to A change or egophony). Abnormal findings can be indicative of increased density in the underlying tissue. Common qualifying descriptors relating to these sounds can be listed as loudness, location, pitch, profusion, and timing.[12] Use of this classification promotes reliability of communication and increases the likelihood of establishing a baseline and documenting change in any patient.

Table 4-3. Categorization of Lung Sounds

Sound	Category
Breath sounds	**Normal** Vesicular: quiet movement of air Bronchovesicular: slightly tubular, louder Bronchial/tracheal: louder, tubular **Abnormal** Decreased: unable to auscultate to appropriate loudness level Absent: unable to auscultate at all Bronchial: heard in inappropriate anatomic location
Adventitious/additional sounds[a]	Coarse crackle: discontinuous, loud, low in pitch, synonomous with coarse rale Fine crackle: discontinuous, quieter, higher in pitch, shorter duration, synonomous with fine rale Wheeze: continuous, high-pitched, long whistling sound, synonomous with sibilant rhonchus Rhonchus: continuous, low-pitched, loud, snoring sound, synonomous with sonorous rhonchus
Voice sounds	Egophony: E to A change; bleating quality indicating consolidation Whispered pectoriloqy: increased articulation of whispered voice sound indicating increased density in underlying lung

a (Definitions from Murphy and Holford.[11])

TESTS AND MEASURES

At the completion of interview and examination, a composite picture of the patient should be coming into focus, to serve as the basis for selecting the appropriate objective tests and measures to better characterize the patient's condition. The most simple and reliable objective tests and measures are positional vital signs, height, and weight. Chronologic recording of these values often provides the basis for deciding when a significant change from baseline indicates the need for more invasive tests or treatment.

Thoracic Imaging

Baseline and serial chest x-ray results provide the physical therapist with essential information regarding the acuity or chronicity of the pulmonary disease process, and, in the acute setting, provide immediate feedback on the patient's response to treatment (e.g., post-treatment lung re-expansion). Although chest x-rays are not specifically diagnostic for many conditions, they can document the following:

1. Local, segmental, or total lung collapse
2. Potential presence of solid or fluid within the lung, circulation, airways, or pleural space
3. Hyperinflation of the lung and change in diaphragmatic position with inspiration/expiration or position change.

Any of these findings, considered within the context of the patient's history and current presentation, may be useful in treatment planning. Other imaging that provides information that may effect the patient includes the ventilation/perfusion scan and chest computerized tomography (CT).

Pulmonary Function Tests

Pulmonary function tests (PFT) include measures of lung volume, air flow, ventilatory muscle strength, and ventilatory muscle endurance. The tests to document these values are interdependent, mostly effort dependent, and provide the information needed to demonstrate ventilatory pump capacity. Each value potentially can be measured in a variety of ways, from a simple, inexpensive, effort-dependent method (water seal spirometry), to an invasive and expensive method (esophageal balloons or plethysmography). Consequently, only the measure and its clinical value will be the focus in this discussion.

Static lung volumes such as tidal volume (Vt), vital capacity (VC), closing volume, and functional residual capacity (FRC) are indicators of (1) the total volume available to the individual (VC) for response to increased oxygen demand, (2) the percentage of the total volume exchanged at rest to meet oxygen demand (Vt), and (3) the amount of volume residing in the system available to participate in gas exchange (FRC and closing volume). A nondiseased man (67 in. tall, 31 years old) with a 4.6 L VC, 2.4 L FRC, and 500 ml Vt is using approximately 10 percent of his VC at rest to perform gas exchange, leaving him with a significant volume of reserve capacity to respond to any increase in oxygen demand. The same man after an auto injury resulting in an incomplete C5–C6 spinal cord injury, left with a 1L VC, 500 ml FRC, and 400 ml Vt, will have significantly less ventilatory reserve and maximum ventilatory capacity to meet any demand for increased oxygen uptake.

Normal values for volume and flow can be reasonably predicted by equations using age, sex, and height reference values.[13–15] Significant reduction in the volume capacity is categorized as restrictive lung disease and is commonly caused by disease that limits lung expansion (e.g., pulmonary fibrosis, mesothelioma) or chest wall motion (e.g., neuromuscular disease, pain, obesity).

Measures of airflow document the volume of gas moved per unit of time. The major factors affecting airflow are the ability to generate muscle force, compliance of the lung and chest wall, and the diameter of the airway. Factors that either increase the ventilatory muscle load, decrease the muscles' ability to generate force, or decrease airway diameter can decrease the rate of air flow. An FVC maneuver can measure the volume of air exhaled over a one- (FEV_1) to three-second period. When calculated as a percentage of the total exhaled volume (FEV_1/FVC), this value indicates the degree of obstruction present. Diseases that constrict the airway (smooth muscle contraction, airway swelling) or obstruct the airway (airway collapse, thick secretions) will increase resistance and reduce flow. These diseases are categorized as obstructive lung diseases.

Measures of volume and flow are most often effort-dependent tests, as they require patient cooperation and coordination. Use of flow–volume loop spirometry for subjects who are less motivated or skilled may increase the reliability of the values.[16] Inability to generate force may also be observed as an inability to perform the maneuver. Simple clinical signs that indicate potential impairment of ventilatory muscle strength and endurance are the inability to sniff or cough or the development of a discoordinated abdominal–thoracic breathing pattern.[17,18]

Diaphragmatic strength and endurance are measured most accurately by invasive procedures to document diaphragmatic force (P_{di}), contraction time, and electromyelogram (EMG) pattern when contracting against a load.[18,19] Clinically it is most feasible to measure maximum inspiratory and expiratory pressure (MIP, MEP) at the mouth with a simple manometer and mouthpiece. MIP and MEP values generated at different lung volumes (residual volume [RV], FRC, total lung capacity [TLC] while seated at rest give an indication of ventilatory muscle strength at varying points on the length–tension curve (see Table 4-4). A wide range of clinical variability has been found when relating these measures to function and that should be carefully considered when relating observed values to predicted functional capacity. Rochester[13] and others[13c] have indicated that the reduction in respiratory muscle strength must be up to 75 percent loss of predicted value before a significant affect on VC is seen. Pathophysiologic factors affecting muscle strength include[20]

Increased resistance to air flow
Elevated minute ventilation due to inefficient gas exchange
Hyperinflation altering muscle length, resulting in
    Reduced ability of diaphragm to generate tension
    Reduced efficiency of diaphragm in generation of negative intrathoracic pressure
    Reduced outward recoil of chest wall
Muscle weakness
Muscle fatigue
Postural abnormalities
Hypoxemia and hypercapnea
Possible pulmonary hypertension

Ventilatory muscle endurance is measured by the muscle's ability to generate and sustain high levels of pressure.[17] Measures such as the tension–time (pressure–time) index of the diaphragm (measure of the contractile force and duration) (TTI_{di}) have then been used to predict onset of fatigue by comparing the load to maximum muscle force over time; however, this measure also requires invasive procedures and complicated calculations not readily available clinically.[22] Because the endurance capacity of the ventilatory pump depends on the intrinsic ventilatory load, the pattern of breathing, respiratory muscle strength, and the force and duration of muscle contraction, it seems logical that stressing the pump to some percentage of its maximum dynamic capacity could potentially demonstrate the endurance range and capacity of the pump. Consequently, measures such as the maximum voluntary ventilation (MVV) and the maximum sustainable ventilatory capacity (MSVC) have proved useful.

The MVV is a function of height, age, and sex, similar to the VC, with the added factors of airway resistance (sGaw) and muscle strength considered. Subjects ventilating at 90 percent or greater of the predicted MVV rapidly demonstrate muscle fatigue.[17] The MSVC has been found to range from 60 to 80 percent of MVV with a mean of 70 percent. Measurement of MVV and MSVC is most easily accomplished using simple spirometry at rest to measure volumes and calculated values (MVV = actual maximum volume breathed for 15 sec. × 4, expressed in liters per minute),[23] or by collecting exhaled gas during exercise. Comparison of actual resting and exercise minute ventilation (RR × Vt = $\dot{V}e$) to MVV provides an indication of ventilatory pump reserve capacity. For example, the 31-year-old man described earlier in this chapter, with a Vt of 500 ml, VC of 4.6 L, and an FEV_1 of 4 L, would have a resting $\dot{V}e$ of 5 L/min (10 × 500 ml). Predicted MVV (35 × FEV_1 = 140 L/min)[23] indicates a ventilatory reserve of 135 L/min to respond to any increased oxygen demand. After the injury described earlier (C5–C6 incomplete cord injury), the patient would conceivably have a similar $\dot{V}e$ (12 × 400 ml = 4.8 L/min) with a decrease in muscle strength (Inspiratory Force (IF) decreased from −110 to −60 mmHg) and decreased pump capacity (predicted MVV = 35 × 1.0 L = 35.0 L/min). Decline in muscle strength and reserve capacity places the patient at risk for decreased ventilatory muscle endurance.

Gas Exchange

Measurements of the efficacy of gas exchange were also risky and expensive to obtain until fairly recently. Blood gas analyzers were first introduced in the late 1950s, literally changing the practice of medicine with their ability to directly measure the oxygen and carbon dioxide pressure within arterial or venous blood.[24] These measures, although incredibly accurate, require an arterial puncture or indwelling catheter, which is most commonly used in the closely monitored setting of the intensive care unit (ICU). Arterial blood gas (ABG) measures remain the gold standard in ICU care for assessing oxygenation and acid-base status (see Table 4-5 and Fig. 4-1 for values). An indwelling catheter provides a manageable port for repeated, immediate measures when

Table 4-4. Typical Values for Ventilatory Muscle Strength Measures

Pressure (cm H_2O)	Lung Volume		
	RV	FRC	TLC
PE max	0	200	240
PI max	−130	−115	0
P_{rs}	−30	0	30
P_{mus} exp	30	200	210
P_{mus} insp	−100	−115	−30

Abbreviations: PE max and PI max, Maximal static respiratory pressures at the mouth; P_{rs}, Respiratory system recoil; P_{mus} exp (PE max − Prs) and P_{mus} insp (PI max − P_{rs}), respiratory muscle pressures; RV, residual volume; FRC, functional residual capacity; TLC, total lung capacity. (Data from Rochester.[18])

necessary and can be used as a line to transduce and monitor arterial pressure. Alveolar–arterial oxygen tension difference (A–aDO_2) can also be calculated from arterial blood to assess the ventilation/perfusion ratio.

Gas analyzers are also commonly used with computer calculations to analyze inhaled and exhaled volumes and estimate diffusing capacity (DLCO), oxygen consumption ($\dot{V}O_2$) and carbon dioxide production (VCO$_2$) (see Table 4-6 for values). The recent technologic development of noninvasive gas monitoring devices (transcutaneous oxygen pressure [PtcO_2] and pulse oximetry) has completely changed clinical practice, providing the ability to rapidly and effectively measure the efficacy of oxygenation in a variety of circumstances. Transcutaneous monitoring of PO$_2$ is very useful in the neonatal population, where rapid changes in oxygen can have dramatic clinical consequences. Disadvantages of this method are risk of skin damage due to the heating element and lack of immediate information when sensor position has to be changed.[24] Similarly, these principles apply to individuals monitored in the ICU or recovery room; therefore, continuous repositioning of patients for treatment might have an effect on accuracy of measurement if the transducer moved.

Table 4-5. Physiologic Values for Oxygen Saturation: Relationship of Transcutaneous Oxygen to Arterial Oxygen

Age Group	PtcO_2 Index (PtcO_2:PaO_2)
Premature	1.14
Newborn	1
Pediatric	0.84
Adult	0.79
Older adult	0.68

Abbreviations: PtcO_2, transcutaneous oxygen pressure; PaO_2, partial arterial pressure of oxygen. (Data from Tremper and Barker.[25])

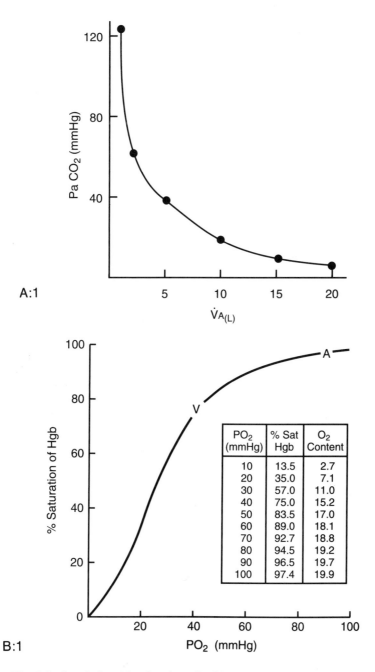

Fig. 4-1. Physiologic relationship of carbon dioxide to alveolar ventilation and of oxygen to hemoglobin in arterial blood. (**A**) The hyperbolic relationship between alveolar ventilation ($\dot{V}_A$) and arterial carbon dioxide tension ($PaCO_2$). (**B**) Oxyhemoglobin dissociation curve: venous (V) and arterial (A) points are indicated. Inset presents partial pressure of oxygen (PO_2), saturation percent of hemoglobin (% Sat Hgb), and oxygen content (O_2), with hemoglobin presumed to be at 15 g/100 ml. (From Tisi,[16] with permission.)

Pulse oximeters do not directly measure oxygen saturation (SaO_2), but observe pulsatile change in light absorption of the blood.[26,27] The accuracy of the measure depends on the amount of oxyhemoglobin in the blood, and this may be altered by the presence of other light absorbers, such as carboxyhemoglobin, in the blood. Advantages of measurement with this device include ease of availability, relative accuracy (95 percent confidence interval of 3 to 5 percent above arterial saturation of 65 percent,[28,29]) and low-risk noninvasive measurement. Its disadvantage is lowered accuracy with motion: a 5 percent change or inaccuracy in saturation can represent a wide range in oxygen tension (Fig. 4-1). Monitoring by oximetry gives immediate gas exchange information to the physical therapist regarding the patient's response to rest, position change, treatment, or activity.

Noninvasive assessment of carbon dioxide or end-tidal carbon dioxide (end-tidal PCO_2) can be measured in the intubated patient during exhaled gas collection or by placing a catheter in the posterior pharynx.[30,31] End-tidal CO_2 approximates PCO_2 (within 4 mmHg) if the subject has well-matched ventilation and perfusion. Unfortunately, with increased physiologic dead space (V_D) and right to left shunt, the measure is less accurate and best used to identify trends.

Measures of $\dot{V}O_2$ and VCO_2 can be performed only by actual measurement and analysis of inhaled and exhaled gas volumes. This requires an intubated patient or a closed ventilation system with a gas analysis computer. Values calculated from actual measures of $\dot{V}O_2$ and VCO_2 can be compared to predicted values for age and sex to demonstrate the aerobic and anaerobic contribution to metabolic activity and to describe both external and internal respiration or gas exchange of an individual (see Table 4-6).

Cardiovascular Measures

Simple and complex cardiovascular assessment skills are essential when establishing a baseline or assessing physical response to activity in a patient with pulmonary impairment. The interrelationship of the cardiac pump, ventilatory pump, and circulation allow the therapist to evaluate the effect of disease or therapeutic measures on either of the systems by monitoring both. A baseline electrocardiogram (ECG) establishes the rate and rhythm of cardiac contraction. An increase or decrease in rate or alteration of rhythm can be reliably assessed by either palpation or ECG. Simultaneous pressure monitoring pro-

Table 4-6. Prediction Equations for Maximum Oxygen Consumption

Gender	Equations
Males	$\dot{V}O_2$ max = 4.2 − 0.032 age L/min (SD ± 0.4)
	$\dot{V}O_2$ max = 60 − 0.55 age ml/kg/min (SD ± 7.5)
Females	$\dot{V}O_2$ max = 2.6 − 0.014 age L/min (SD ± 0.4)
	$\dot{V}O_2$ max = 48 − 0.37 age ml/kg/min (SD ± 7.0)

(Data from Jones et al.[39])

Table 4-7. Normal Resting Values for Blood Pressure

Age (years)	Systolic Pressure (mmHg)	Systolic Pressure (kPa)	Diastolic Pressure (mmHg)	Diastolic Pressure (kPa)
Men				
65–69	143	19.1	83	11.1
85–89	145	19.3	79	10.5
95–106	145	19.3	78	10.4
Women				
65–69	154	20.5	85	11.3
85–89	154	20.5	82	10.9
95–106	149	19.9	81	10.8

Abbreviation: kPa, kilopascals.
(From Shephard,[49] with permission.)

vides additional information. Normal systolic and diastolic blood pressure response to changes of age,[32] position,[33] and activity[34] are all well documented. Knowledge of baseline values and ranges for normal change provides an accurate basis for determining the implications and consequences of observed actual values (see Tables 4-7 through 4-9).

Invasive central pressure monitoring in an ICU or recovery room setting can be used to document response to treatment and corroborate other examination findings. For example, the ICU patient in respiratory failure with a past history of myocardial infarction who experienced an increase in coarse crackles, respiratory rate, and heart rate with arterial hypoxemia (see Table 4-10) during Trendelenburg positioning would be more safely monitored and managed with central pressure monitoring, ECG, and oximetry. Cardiovascular monitoring is an integral part of pulmonary assessment.

Posture, Strength, and Range of Motion

Documentation of posture requires the skill of observation in concert with knowledge of baseline standards and common groupings for classification of abnormality. Kendall has classified common postural abnormalities and, with Sahrmann, grouped individuals in terms of length–tension muscle imbalance.[35]

Table 4-8. Physiologic Response to Activity: Oxygen and Ventilation Requirements

Activity	$\dot{V}O_2$ (L/min)	$\dot{V}e$ (L/min)
Basal	0.25	6.3
Sitting at desk	0.35	8.8
Walking slowly (<3 kph)	0.6	15
Getting dressed, light work (seated)	0.7	17.5
Walking briskly (5 kph)	1.0	25
Climbing stairs	1.6	40
Running, shoveling snow	2.0	50
Cross-country skiing	3.5	90

(Data from Rochester.[18])

Table 4-9. Incremental Treadmill Cardiopulmonary Exercise Protocol and Normal Response

Stage	Speed/Grade (mph/%)	METs	HR (bpm)	SBP/DBP (mmHg)	$\dot{V}e$ (L/min)	Vt (ml)	RR (bpm)
1	1.0/0	2.6	96 ± 15	140 ± 13/96 ± 8	18 ± 6	1153 ± 417	17 ± 4
2	1.5/0	3.1	98 ± 14	141 ± 12/93 ± 8	20 ± 5	1162 ± 450	19 ± 4
3	2.0/3.5	3.8	104 ± 13	145 ± 13/91 ± 7	24 ± 7	1270 ± 368	20 ± 4
4	2.0/7.0	4.7	110 ± 13	150 ± 13/87 ± 8	29 ± 9	1388 ± 394	22 ± 4
5	2.0/10.5	5.4	118 ± 14	155 ± 13/92 ± 11	33 ± 9	1468 ± 405	24 ± 3
6	3.0/7.5	6.2	126 ± 13	159 ± 21/87 ± 8	40 ± 12	1628 ± 456	25 ± 4
7	3.0/10.0	6.9	135 ± 15	168 ± 19/88 ± 9	46 ± 14	1776 ± 502	27 ± 6
8	3.0/12.5	7.9	144 ± 15	166 ± 19/91 ± 11	52 ± 17	1921 ± 502	28 ± 7
9	3.0/15.0	8.7	155 ± 14	169 ± 25/88 ± 10	61 ± 19	2153 ± 681	29 ± 7
10	3.4/14.0	9.2	162 ± 15	179 ± 21/86 ± 14	72 ± 25	2261 ± 700	33 ± 10

Abbreviations: HR, heart rate; METs, metabolic equivalent (1 MET = 3.5 ml/min/kg O_2 uptake); SBP/DBP, systolic and diastolic blood pressure; $\dot{V}e$, minute ventilation; Vt, tidal volume; RR, respiratory rate; bpm, beats per minute.
(Data from Weber et al.[51])

These groupings are useful to establish a baseline for treatment approach, particularly when incorporating breathing exercises and functional activities with goals to reduce pulmonary impairment.

Strength measures for ventilatory muscles have been described previously in this chapter. The remaining skeletal muscles of the limbs and trunk are measured and graded manually according to conventional scales of either Kendall and McCreary[35] or Daniels and Worthingham.[36] Minimum range of motion (ROM) documentation should include measurement of all joints with obvious and functional limitations. Simple observation will not be sufficiently accurate to demonstrate change after therapeutic intervention. Miller has described nicely the limitations of "eyeballing" joint measures and the reliability and validity problems with established norms.[37] Given these drawbacks, ROM changes in the upper extremity, for example, can be dramatic in terms of functional gains after an integrated posture and breathing exercise therapeutic program. The pulmonary impaired population in general, and particularly those who are severely limited and deconditioned, respond well to general conditioning focused on mobility and strength.

Table 4-10. Central Cardiovascular Pressure Values

Value	mmHg
Right atrium mean	−1–+7
Right ventricle	
Systolic	15–25
End diastolic	0–8
Pulmonary artery	
Systolic	15–25
Diastolic	8–15
Mean	10–20
Pulmonary capillary wedge	
Mean	6–12

FUNCTIONAL ASSESSMENT

All assessment tests and measures described previously have predominantly taken place with the patient at rest. Considering that the goal of rehabilitation is to return the patient to the "highest functional capacity,"[38] given the patient's level of impairment and disability, some measures must document baseline and maximum functional capacity to safely and accurately plan treatment and demonstrate improvement with therapy. Additionally, some patients will present with "normal" values at rest, but exhibit abnormal characteristics only during activity. Cardiopulmonary exercise testing (CPX) places performance demands on all systems participating in the oxygen uptake and delivery required to produce musculoskeletal movement (cardiovascular, pulmonary, musculoskeletal). Observation and measurement of exercise response from rest through gradually increasing workloads can implicate or eliminate each system as a participant in the impairment of movement and provide a basis for directing treatment.

Exercise Test Protocols

There are many standardized test protocols available in the current literature for the assessment of cardiopulmonary response to exercise.[39] Most are designed to incrementally and progressively increase oxygen demand by increasing work performed by the large muscle groups of the lower extremities while walking or cycling. Some clinicians have acknowledged the wide range of physical performance ability in the population and adapted exercise test protocols to meet the needs of specifically limited populations (e.g., walk tests for chronic obstructive pulmonary disease [COPD] patients or upper extremity exercise protocols for paraplegic individuals).[40,41] This concept, applied broadly, allows the physical therapist flexibility in the design of any exercise assessment situation. A CPX test can then theoretically occur during any standardized activity where the intensity, duration, workload, and response are controlled and measured.

Standardized protocols, such as the Bruce or Balke, are excellent for the general population who do not exhibit signs and symptoms of impairment at rest and have some reserve exercise capacity, yet complain of fatigue and severe dyspnea after going up two flights of stairs carrying groceries[39,42] (see Table 4-11). These protocols control the intensity of workload by setting speed and incline on a treadmill for timed segments. Large numbers of individuals have performed these tests, creating an accurate database for comparison of normal and abnormal response. However, stage I of the Bruce Protocol requires the subject to walk at 1.7 mph up a 10 percent grade on a treadmill. This may not be possible for a 75-year-old patient with a right hemiplegia or a 55-year-old COPD patient with a permanent tracheostomy who is mechanically ventilated at night and needs a functional activity program to increase endurance capacity. An exercise assessment is essential to determine the maximum functional ability and sources of impairment for these patients and provides the essential basis for treatment program design.

Selection of the appropriate protocol is based on the findings of the physical examination and objective tests and measures previously described. Subjects with lower extremity impairment, dyspnea, or angina at rest may require either an upper extremity, seated CPX, or low-level walk test (Table 4-11). Test performance for these patients may also require an ambulatory assistive device or the use of oxygen during testing. Maximum performance will be documented as having been performed with the additional support. By test protocol adaptation, the maximum exercise capacity of a paraplegic who experiences angina when propelling a manual wheelchair can be documented, as it can for the obese, sedentary, smoking 55-year-old who complains of dyspnea with stair climbing.

Variables to be considered during protocol selection for each test include[46]

1. Exercise mode (walking, pedaling, or cranking)
2. Setting and environmental conditions (e.g., intensive care unit, exercise lab, home setting, community program, etc.)
3. Patient's condition and goals (e.g., weaning from the ventilator or reducing risk of coronary artery disease progression after coronary bypass surgery)

A protocol is selected that begins exercise at a workload that the subject can perform long enough to achieve steady state (2 to 6 min) and then progress through incremental increases in work that will eventually elicit maximum performance. Workload can be added in a continuous, progressive fashion, as in the Bruce Protocol for subjects with a moderate to large exercise and reserve capacity. Workload can be increased intermittently if a subject is unable to

Table 4-11. Exercise Test Protocols

Test	Protocol
Bruce[43]	Treadmill test: four progressive 3-min stages, increasing speed and grade (1.7 mph, 10% grade; 2.5 mph, 12% grade; 3.4 mph, 14% grade; 4.2 mph, 16% grade)
Balke[44]	Treadmill test: 2-min progressive stages, increasing grade by 2.5% while speed is kept constant at 2 mph
Low-Level 2 Stage Test[29c]	Walk/pedal test: stage I, set treadmill/ergometer at lowest possible speed, grade, load. Subject walks, rides, cranks for 6 min, attempting to achieve steady state. Subjects who quickly achieve steady state by 3–4 min will be progressed into a second stage without rest. Subjects who are unable to achieve 6 min or steady state do not progress. Stage II used to elicit maximum function in remaining subjects.
Timed-Walk Test[45]	Hallway walk test: subject instructed to walk as far and as fast as possible in time allotted (3, 6, 12 min); clinical signs monitored, total distance documented
Ergometer Test[39]	Specific workload set: subject rides or cranks at steady rpm for preset time (2–3 min); workload increase determined by response to previous stage

perform more than 4 to 6 min of activity at once. By allowing the subject to return to resting level, additional information can be gained through performance of a second stage of the activity (e.g., dyspnea alone may prevent progression at stage I; stage II may produce MVV and ventilatory pump impairment). The goal of testing is to monitor response to activity and determine systemic limitations to performance that can be treated with medication or training. Because training effects are activity specific, the exercise test should also document pretraining maximum values in the specific activity where training improvements are necessary and will be demonstrated.

MONITORING RESPONSE TO ACTIVITY

Measuring and interpreting an individual's response to activity includes tracking the magnitude of change in each of the physiologic parameters observed and documented at rest. The change required for each incremental increase in workload will be compared to the resting level and the predicted maximum of an individual, given age, sex, and medical history. Large-population cross-sectional studies have provided data for age-predicted changes in resting and maximum values of heart rate (HR), blood pressure (BP), RR, $\dot{V}e$, and $\dot{V}O_2$.[40,47–49] Other studies have cited the normal range of change expected for any given increase in workload (Tables 4-10 and 4-12). The wide range of predicted response is generally intended to accommodate for age, sex, size, and condition differences. Although these values are useful as guidelines, they need to be applied with care, as the validity of broad ranges decreases as the extremes are approached.

Physiologic response parameters that are simplest and least expensive to monitor in any clinical situation include heart rate and rhythm, BP, RR,

Table 4-12. Suggested Normal Values for Cycle Exercise Testing in Middle-aged Men[a]

Measure	Value
$\dot{V}O_2$ max	90% of predicted treadmill $\dot{V}O_2$ max[b] using ideal body weight
Anaerobic threshold	>40% of predicted $\dot{V}O_2$ max
Breathing reserve (MVV − $\dot{V}e$ max)	>15 L/min
Breathing pattern	Vt < VC; RR < 60 breaths per minute
ABG at maximal exercise	
PAO_2	> 80 mmHg
$P(A–a)O_2$	< 35 mmHg
V_D:Vt	< 0.30
$P(a–ET)CO_2$	< 0 mmHg

Abbreviations: $\dot{V}O_2$ max, maximum oxygen uptake; RR, respiratory rate; Vt, tidal volume; VC, vital capacity; MVV, maximum voluntary ventilation; ABG, arterial blood gases; PAO_2, alveolar oxygen partial pressure; $P(A–a)O_2$, partial pressure of alveolar–arterial oxygen tension difference; V_D: Vt, ratio of dead space to tidal volume; $P(a–ET)CO_2$, alveolar–end tidal carbon dioxide tension difference.

[a] (From Sue and Hansen,[54] with permission.)
[b] (Data from Bruce and McDonough.[43])

breathing pattern, SaO_2, and symptoms. Heart rate and rhythm can be palpated or more reliably recorded by ECG. Rapid rise in heart rate or development of arrhythmia with minimal activity may indicate cardiac impairment along a range from deconditioning to pathology (Table 4-13). Similarly, rapid rise in BP or fall in SBP with increasing workloads can indicate either cardiac or circulatory incompetence.[50,51] Respiratory rate and breathing pattern are useful indicators of ventilatory pump capability and, when evaluated with SaO_2, provide a basis for assessing gas exchange. A rapid rise in RR may signal decreased lung–thorax compliance and increased resistance to flow, while a discoordinated breathing pattern highlights an increased work of breathing (WOB) and may indicate

Table 4-13. Physiologic Measures as Indicators of Impairment

Indicator	Measures
Ventilatory pump impairment	Achievement of predicted MVV, inability to maintain adequate MIP and/or development of discoordinated breathing, RR of 50–70, dyspnea
Minute ventilation ($\dot{V}e$)	$35 \times FEV_1$ (actual) is rough MVV estimate. Ventilation reaching or exceeding this value at minimum exercise intensities means poor probability for exercise conditioning.
Maximum inspiratory pressure (mouth)	Critical level, 40–60 cm H_2O. Below these values, ventilatory muscle training may need to precede or accompany exercise conditioning
Increased flow resistance	Development of bronchospasm or mucus mobilization, decreased FEV_1, change in ventilatory pattern and muscle use, dyspnea.
Gas exchange impairment	Decreasing SaO_2 or PaO_2, increasing $PaCO_2$, dizziness, nausea, dyspnea, ECG abnormality
Oxygenation	Tolerable range for rest/exercise: $SaO_2 > 99\%$ to 85%, $PaO_2 > 104$ mmHg $- (.42 \times age)$ to 60 mmHg. Inability to maintain within tolerable range indicates need for supplemental oxygen
Cardiac impairment	Rapid inappropriate increase in heart rate, no increase in heart rate with increase in workload, no increase or significant decrease in blood pressure with increase in workload, ECG abnormality, dyspnea, angina
Heart rate	$(220 - age)$ up to age 60. After, 60 men plateau at 170, women, at 160. Ability to reach 85% maximum predicted or greater without limitation means good probability for exercise conditioning
Deconditioning	Appropriate cardiopulmonary response that quickly reaches predicted maximum cardiac values, symptom limitations (e.g., fear, weak extremities, lack of coordination)

Abbreviations: MVV, maximum voluntary ventilation; FEV_1, forced expiratory volume in one second; SaO_2, oxygen saturation; PaO_2, partial pressure of arterial oxygen; RR, respiratory rate.

impending respiratory failure.[52,53] Decrease in SaO_2 has not been a normal finding in activity, despite decline in PO_2 with age.

More invasive and equipment-intensive monitoring can provide a clearer picture of maximum exercise capacity and specific system impairment. Monitoring of heart rate, rhythm, and pattern by ECG will demonstrate cardiac changes associated with ischemia. Use of a closed ventilation system with a pneumotachograph, gas analyzer, computer, and indwelling arterial catheter provides breath-to-breath analysis of gas flow and concentration. Data collected throughout exercise and calculations made from values monitored with such a system can yield information such as $\dot{V}O_2$ max, $\dot{V}$e max, HR max, oxygen pulse, and anaerobic threshold.

Sue and Hansen studied a group of 77 current and former shipyard workers in an attempt to monitor most exercise response values and compare them to predicted norms in a nondiseased population.[54] The investigators studied a population of 257 men with physical examination, CXR, ECG, PFT, and exercise tests to eliminate those with any history or evidence of heart disease, lung disease, chest wall disease, neuromuscular or musculoskeletal abnormality, malignancy, cirrhosis, or poorly controlled diabetes. Subjects were not eliminated for obesity, hypertension or smoking. A summary of the results of monitoring these subjects during cycle exercise indicates that monitoring exercise response can categorize individuals into normal or pathologic groups by observing the components of the cardiovascular or pulmonary system (Tables 4-10 and 4-12).

Additional data can be collected by quantifying subjective or symptomatic response to exercise. By documenting the workload at which dyspnea, chest pressure, or jaw pain occurs, a pattern may be established that objectively records onset of angina. Use of an interval category or visual analog scale to measure dyspnea aids in linking this symptom to a specific cardiovascular, pulmonary, or musculoskeletal indicator of fatigue or failure.[20,55] (Table 4-14 and Fig. 4-2). Recording of all values at 2-minute intervals throughout the test pinpoints the workload and time that an abnormality develops in each system. Simultaneous tracking of symptoms completes the picture, for example, illustrating onset of pain, nausea, or dyspnea at the same time ST segment depression and rapid HR rate rise occur.

Interpreting Exercise Response

Interpreting the results of a CPX requires summary of all data elicited during both static and dynamic phases of the examination. Comparing values that are within normal limits at rest with abnormalities elicted during exercise indicates that any existing pathologic process has currently impaired only the reserve capacity of the individual. The earlier the onset of impairment in exercise (decrease in maximum capacity or achievement of maximum capacity at minimum workload), the greater the functional limitation an abnormality has produced. Impairment is assessed by clustering of values related to each system (see Table 4-13).

Table 4-14. Quantification of Dyspnea: Borg Category Scale

Rank	Definition
0	Nothing at all
0.5	Very, very slight (just noticeable)
1	Very slight
2	Slight
3	Moderate
4	Somewhat severe
5	Severe
6	
7	Very severe
8	
9	Very, very severe (almost maximal)
10	Maximal

(From Borg,[55] with permission.)

Cardiovascular impairment, such as hypertension or myocardial ischemia, will be indicated by rapidly increasing or falling blood pressure, abnormal heart rate, response to increased workload, change in ECG, breath sounds, heart sounds, and symptoms such as fatigue and dyspnea at low levels of activity. Ventilatory pump impairment may be observed at rest with use of accessory muscles and supraclavicular retraction. Secondary findings can include an increased RV and decreased VC, with an FEV_1 of less than 30 percent, predicted

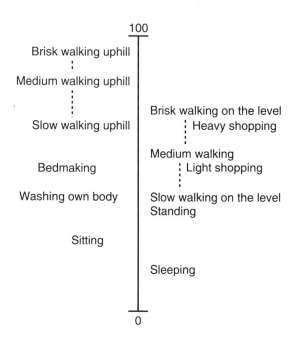

Fig. 4-2. Oxygen cost diagram. (From McGavin et al.,[56] with permission.)

by PFT. A predicted MVV of 35L/min (FEV$_1$ × 35) that is reached during the first four minutes of low-level exercise (treadmill [TM] walking at 1.5 mph, 0 percent grade) as the patient develops a discoordinated breathing pattern and complains of a grade IX dyspnea completes the picture.[55] Additional values strengthening this interpretation would include significantly decreased inspiratory and expiratory force measures.

Although both impairments described above include the common symptom of dyspnea, the other parameters described differ. Kanarek and Hand have pointed out that despite substantial reduction of lung function in some cardiac patients, these individuals are so limited by cardiovascular factors that at maximum exercise they leave unused a significant portion of their ventilatory reserve.[57] This thinking provides the basis for much of the interpretation of exercise response; knowing or predicting the maximum capacity of each component of the system provides a baseline for evaluating response as a percentage of maximum. Patients who achieve maximum in a given monitoring parameter (HR, RR, BP, MVV, dyspnea) or cross into an abnormal/pathologic range or pattern (SaO$_2$ < 88 percent, IF < −50 mmHg, discoordinated breathing) must be considered as having used all the reserve capacity available in that system. This, then, is the component or system most responsible for contributing to and potentially producing the impairment that limits function.

The interrelationship of variables between systems increases the complexity of this process. Patients who have been acutely ill and supine for prolonged periods clearly become deconditioned (see Ch. 8). The process of deconditioning may then mask or override other cardiovascular or pulmonary systemic impairments. However, once the deconditioning process has been treated with training, it is possible to "condition" an individual's cardiovascular system to the point past cardiovascular impairment. Exercise beyond that level, for example, may reveal a ventilatory impairment to further conditioning.

The National Heart, Lung, and Blood Institute (NHLBI) convened in 1988 to discuss the assessment of respiratory impairment in pulmonary disease.[58] Participants agreed that physical examination and lung function tests were essential for establishing the presence and type of respiratory disease. However, they concluded that increasing demand for ventilation and gas exchange with exercise would be more effective at highlighting functional abnormality associated with respiratory limitation. Finally, they also concluded that exercise tests remain difficult to interpret and an area requiring further research. Because non-respiratory factors (cardiovascular and neuromuscular abnormalities, deconditioning and obesity) often contribute to performance, these may have relatively greater or lesser effect on a given individual, making interpretation difficult.

SUMMARY

The physical therapy examination and assessment is directed toward eliciting the signs and symptoms of pathology that produce impairment and subsequent disability.[58] Grimby cites examples such as cough, sputum, and breathlessness that fall into the respiratory impairment category. If unrelieved, these impairments may have functional consequences, such as inability to walk rapidly, climb stairs, or participate in some forms of ADL. These limitations fall within the category of disability. Therefore, the goal of any examination is to identify the impairments that, if treated, will reduce or prevent physical disability.

REFERENCES

1. World Health Organization: The First Ten Years of the World Health Organization. Geneva, World Health Organization, 1958
2. Nagi S: Some conceptual issues in disability and rehabilitation. In Sussman M (ed): Sociology and Rehabilitation. American Sociological Association, Washington, D.C., 1965
3. American Medical Association Committee on Medical Rating of Physical Impairment: Guidelines to the evaluation of permanent impairment. JAMA, 1958
4. Jette AM: State of the art in functional status assessment. In Rothstein JM (ed): Measurement in Physical Therapy. Churchill Livingstone, New York, 1985
5. Loudon RG: The lung exam. Clin Chest Med 8:265, 1987
6. Nebnhanni T, Michel TH, Zadai CC: Reliability of chest wall excursion measurement. Phys Ther, in press, 1992
7. Lareau M, Lareau D: Reliability of auscultation among chest physical therapists in a common terminology. Unpublished thesis project.
8. Tretter SM, Dueker JA: Reliability of a method for measurement of the infrasternal angle (abstract). Phys Ther 66:753, 1986
9. Auenbrugger L: Inventum novum ex percussione thoracis humani. Trattner, Vienna, 1761
10. Laennec RTH: A Treatise on the Disease of the Chest. Hafner, New York, 1962
11. Murphy RLH, Holford SK: Lung Sounds. Basics of Respiratory Disease 8:4, 1980
12. Loudon RG: The lung exam. Clin Chest Med 8:265, 1987
13. Lebowitz MD, Knudson RJ, Burrows B et al: Significance of intraindividual changes in maximum expiratory flow volume and peak expiratory flow measurements. Chest 81:566, 1982
14. Knudson RJ, Slatin RL, Lebowitz MD et al: The maximum expiration in flow–volume curve: normal standards, variability and effects of age. Am Rev Respir Dis 113:587, 1976
15. Nickerson BJ, Leman RJ, Gerdes CB et al: Within-subject variability and percent change for significance of spirometry in normal subjects and patients with cystic fibrosis. Am Rev Respir Dis 122:859, 1980
16. Tisi G: Pulmonary Physiology in Clinical Medicine. 2nd Ed. Williams & Wilkins, Baltimore, 1983
17. Roussos C, Fixley M, Gross D et al: Fatigue of inspiratory muscles and their synergistic behavior. J Appl Physiol 46:897, 1979
18. Rochester DF: Tests of respiratory muscle function. Clin Chest Med 9:249, 1988
19. Laporta D, Grassino A: Assessment of transdiaphragmatic pressure in humans. J Appl Physiol 58:1,469, 1985
20. Sweer L, Zwillich CW: Dyspnea in the patient with chronic obstructive pulmonary disease. Clin Chest Med 11:417, 1990

21. Gal TJ, Goldberg SK: Relationship between respiratory muscle strength and vital capacity during partial curarization in awake subjects. Anesthesiol 54:141, 1981
22. Bellemare F, Grassino A: Effect of pressure and timing of contraction on human diaphragm fatigue. J Appl Physiol 53:1190, 1982
23. Cherniack RM: Pulmonary Function Testing. WB Saunders, Philadelphia, 1977
24. Wiedemann HP, McCarthy K: Noninvasive monitoring of oxygen and carbon dioxide. Clin Chest Med 10:239, 1989
25. Tremper KK, Barker SJ: Transcutaneous oxygen measurement: experimental studies and adult applications. Int Anesthesiol Clin 25:67, 1987
26. Huch A, Huch R, Konig V et al: Limitations of pulse oximetry (letter). Lancet 2:357, 1988
27. New W: Pulse oximetry. J Clin Monit 2:126, 1985
28. Ries AL: Oximetry—know thy limits. Chest 91:316, 1987
29. Ries AL, Farrow JT, Clausen JL: Accuracy of two ear oximeters at rest and during exercise in pulmonary patients. Am Rev Respir Dis 132:685, 1985
30. Rebuck AS, Chapman KR: Measurement and monitoring of exhaled carbon dioxide. In Nothomovitz ML, Cherniack NS (eds): Noninvasive Respiratory Monitoring. Churchill Livingstone, New York, 1986
31. Smith TC, Marini JJ: Noninvasive blood gas monitoring: options and limitations. Pulmonary and Critical Care Update 2:1, 1986
32. Wei JY: Cardiovascular anatomic and physiologic changes with age. Topics in Ger Rehab 2:10, 1986
33. Weisfeldt ML (ed): The Aging Heart. Raven Press, New York, 1980
34. Raven PB, Mitchell J: The effect of aging on the cardiovascular response to dynamic and static exercise. In Weisfeldt ML (ed): The Aging Heart. Raven Press, New York, 1980
35. Kendall FP, McCreary EK: Muscles—Testing and Function. Williams & Wilkins, Baltimore, 1983
36. Daniels, Worthingham C: Muscle Testing. Techniques of Manual Examination. 3rd Ed. WB Saunders, Philadelphia, 1972
37. Miller PJ: Assessment of joint motion. In Rothstein J (ed): Measurement in Physical Therapy. Churchill Livingstone, New York, 1985
38. Official American Thoracic Society statement: Pulmonary rehabilitation. Am Rev Respir Dis 124:663, 1981
39. Jones NL, Campbell EJM, Edwards RHT et al: Clinical Exercise Testing. WB Saunders, Philadelphia, 1982
40. Zadai CC: Rehabilitation of the patient with chronic obstructive disease. In Irwin SC, Tecklin JS (eds): Cardiopulmonary Physical Therapy. 2nd Ed. CV Mosby, St. Louis, 1990
41. Sheffield LT, Roitman D: Stress testing methodology. In Sonnenblick EH, Lesch M (eds): Exercise in Heart Disease. Grune & Stratton, New York, 1977
42. Kavanagh T: Exercise and coronary artery disease. In Basmajian JV, Wolf S (eds): Therapeutic Exercise. 5th Ed. Williams & Williams, Baltimore, 1990
43. Bruce RA, McDonough JR: Stress testing in screening for cardiovascular disease. Bull NY Acad Med 45:1,288, 1969
44. Nagle FJ, Balke B, Naughton JP: Gradational step tests for assessing work capacity. J Appl Physiol 20:745, 1965
45. McGavin CR, Gupta SP, McHardy GJ: 12-minute walk test. Br Med J 1:822, 1976
46. Zadai CC: Exercise testing and training for the pulmonary impaired patient. In Basmajian JV, Wolf S (eds): Therapeutic Exercise. 5th Ed. Williams & Williams, Baltimore, 1990

47. American College of Sports Medicine: Guidelines for Graded Exercise Testing and Exercise Prescription. Lea & Febiger, Philadelphia, 1975

48. Irwin SC, Tecklin JS: Cardiopulmonary Physical Therapy. 2nd Ed. CV Mosby, St. Louis, 1990

49. Shephard RJ: Physical Activity and Aging. 2nd Ed. Aspen, Rockville, MD, 1987

50. Irwin SC: Cardiac rehabilitation for the geriatric patient. Topics in Ger Rehab 2:44, 1986

51. Weber KT, Janicki JS, McElroy PA et al: Concepts and applications of cardiopulmonary exercise testing. Chest 93:843, 1988

52. Pourriat JL, Lamberto CH, Hoang PH et al: Diaphragmatic fatigue and breathing pattern during weaning from mechanical ventilation in COPD patients. Chest 90:703, 1986

53. Cohen CA, Zaglebaum G, Gross D et al: Clinical manifestations of inspiratory muscle fatigue. Am J Med 73:308, 1982

54. Sue DY, Hansen JE: Normal values in adults during exercise testing. Clin Chest Med 5(1):89, 1984

55. Borg G: Psychophysical basis of perceived exertion. Med Sci Sports Exer 14:377, 1982

56. McGavin CR, Artvinli M, Naoe H, McHardy GJR: Dyspnea disability and distance walked: comparison of estimates of exercise performance in respiratory disease. Br Med J 2:241, 1978

57. Kanarek DJ, Hand RW: The response of cardiac and pulmonary disease to exercise testing. Clin Chest Med 5:181, 1984

58. Becklake M, Rodarte JR, Kalica AR: Scientific issues in the assessment of respiratory impairment. Am Rev Respir Dis 137:1,505, 1981

5 | Body Positioning

Jocelyn Ross
Elizabeth Dean

The function of the cardiopulmonary system is position dependent: gravity influences the mechanics of the system and is a significant determinant of the distribution of ventilation ($\dot{V}e$) and perfusion ($\dot{Q}$). Although the therapeutic use of body positioning has been integrated into physical therapy practice, the application has been largely limited to effecting secretion clearance.[1-5] There has been less emphasis on the use of body positioning to address all aspects of O_2 transport.[6-8] It is well established that the heart, lungs, and vasculature form a highly integrated unit that effects gas exchange between the atmosphere and cells, and that each step of the oxygen cascade[9] must be considered in clinical interventions designed to optimize tissue oxygenation.[6,10-12] Thus, this chapter discusses the physiologic effects of positioning on O_2 transport, the influence of confounding factors, and the implications for physical therapy practice, within the context of a problem-solving approach to positioning management of patients.

OXYGEN TRANSPORT IN THE UPRIGHT POSITION

The upright lung is the standard position used for lung function testing and for determining the effect of altered body position on mechanics, lung volumes, and the distribution of $\dot{V}e$ and $\dot{Q}$.[9,13] In this position, gravity acts along the vertical axis of the body to exert its greatest influence on the distribution of $\dot{V}e$ and $\dot{Q}$, while mechanical compression of the cardiopulmonary unit is minimal.[12,14]

Pulmonary Mechanics

In the upright position, the rib cage assumes its greatest anteroposterior diameter. In this position, the inspiratory intercostals and scalenes are lengthened, while the abdomen falls away from the diaphragm, so that these fibers are

79

shortened.[15] The neural drive to the diaphragm is increased in sitting to offset the shortened position and the resultant decrease in force generated in this position.[16,17] The attendant tonic abdominal muscle activity (related to the distending pressure of the abdomen) has been considered as a mechanism for counteracting the caudal displacement of the diaphragm.[18] This increased respiratory muscle work is likely to be compensated for by the increased mechanical advantage.

Position-induced changes in the chest wall have been related to the observation that resting tidal volume (Vt) is accomplished predominantly by rib cage motion in the upright position.[19] The effect of posture on lung volumes—with the upright lung as the reference position—is well known, having been the subject of some classic studies on healthy individuals.[14,20] Table 5-1 contains representative data from Kaneko et al.[14] on the effect of posture on lung volume and is discussed in sections specific to each position.

Cardiovascular Mechanics

The primary hemodynamic effect of a change in posture is a redistribution of venous volume, with secondary changes in ventricular filling, stroke volume (SV), and thus $\dot{Q}$.[21] The physiologic response to a change in posture is largely determined by the magnitude of the volume shift. In the upright position, the cardiovascular system must work harder to maintain its $\dot{Q}$, due to the significant decrease in venous return.[22] A 700 ml fluid shift from the upper to lower body occurs, wherein the majority of the blood volume is displaced from the intrathoracic cardiovascular compartments.[23] In standing, 70 percent of the total blood volume is below the level of the heart, and is contained in the highly compliant venous system,[24] which is able to maintain blood pressure during a large loss of circulating volume, but is less effective in dealing with orthostatic stress. However, mechanisms inherent in the venous system structure enhance its limited ability to deal with that stress. As blood pools in the veins during standing, the veins become stiffer and thus oppose further filling. In addition, the walls of the veins below the heart are thicker, and thus less compliant, than those above the heart. Further, the venous valves slow the displacement of blood from the thorax to the dependent veins on assumption of the upright posture.[25] As the dependent veins fill, the valves are progressively forced open, so that the blood is displaced in several stages. The significance of these valves is exemplified in individuals with valve incompetence or absence, who suffer from severe orthostatic intolerance without the use of counteractive measures such as elastic stockings.[26] Even with these mechanisms, the circulation is able only to tolerate an active upright posture, where venous return is assisted by the powerful pumping action of the leg muscles. These muscles work in combination with the valves, which prevent backflow between contractions, and are able to generate 90 mmHg of driving force.[27] It has been shown that minimal activity in the antigravity muscles can decrease the amount of pooling in the legs, but

Table 5-1. Physical Characteristics, Lung Volumes,[a] and Vertical Lung Length[b] at Total Lung Capacity

Subject	Age (years)	Height (cm)	Weight (kg)	D (cm)	Seated			Supine			Prone		
					TLC	FRC	RV	TLC	FRC	RV	TLC	FRC	RV
HD	31	177	79	19	7.06	3.59	1.56	6.50	2.60	1.30	6.58	2.78	1.38
GD	26	180	83	18	6.09	2.79	1.58	5.92	1.99	1.39	5.77	2.58	1.50
DT	32	167	73	20	5.65	2.81	1.25	5.37	1.94	1.31	5.49	2.06	1.34

Subject	Age (years)	Height (cm)	Weight (kg)	D (cm)	Seated			Right Lateral			Left Lateral		
					TLC	FRC	RV	TLC	FRC	RV	TLC	FRC	RV
GO	27	168	56	27	5.78	3.08	1.78	5.61	2.83	1.81			
GA	34	170	65	27	6.15	3.00	1.70	5.75	2.65	1.41			
KK	34	166	59	27	5.33	2.32	1.28	5.20	2.42	1.30	5.27	2.52	1.46
MW	34	181	81	29	7.33	3.03	1.82				7.20	2.86	1.70
BS	32	173	72	25	5.90	3.00	1.50				5.65	2.15	1.45

Abbreviations: D, vertical lung length; TLC, total lung capacity; FRC, functional residual capacity; RV, residual volume.
[a] Lung volumes were determined by the closed-circuit helium method and are expressed in liters.
[b] Vertical lung length was determined with radiographs taken in each posture studied in each subject, in the first three subjects being measured when they were supine, and in the remaining five when they were in the right or left lateral position. (From Kaneko et al.,[14] with permission.)

modest muscle activity in a static position is needed to restore central venous volume.[28,29] The respiratory system also acts as a pump during inspiration, where the intrathoracic pressure becomes more negative and thereby assists venous return.[30] In addition to those responses to the upright position, central and peripheral regulatory reflex mechanisms maintain homeostasis as discussed in Chapter 8.[21,23] The net result of these mechanisms in quiet standing is a 5 mmHg fall in right atrial pressure; a 40 percent decrease in SV with a compensatory increase in heart rate (HR), resulting in a 20 percent decrease in Q̇; and little change in mean pressure due to compensatory vasoconstriction.[31] Representative values for hemodynamic parameters and left ventricular performance in supine and sitting positions are shown in Table 5-2. Although these changes challenge the circulation to maintain Q̇, they have a positive impact on the work of the heart in the upright position. Langou et al.[32] observed a decrease both in left ventricular chamber size (thus, ventricular wall stress) and myocardial O_2 demand in dogs on assumption of the upright position. They suggested that the decrease in myocardial demand in the upright position was responsible for previous observations that nitroglycerin has a greater effect when administered to patients in the upright position.[33] In addition, compression of the cardiac chambers seen during horizontal positioning is not of significance in the upright position.[34,35] Thus, despite the increased orthostatic stress on the cardiovascular system in the upright position (see Ch. 8), there is less mechanical compression of the heart and a lower myocardial O_2 demand.

Table 5-2. Direct Hemodynamic Measurements,[a] Left Ventricular Dimensions, and Performance[b] in Normal Subjects at Rest

Parameter	Supine	Sitting
Heart rate (beats/min)	73 ± 4	84 ± 4
Pressure (mmHg)		
Brachial artery	96 ± 3	99 ± 4
Systolic	130 ± 5	132 ± 5
Diastolic	76 ± 3	82 ± 3
Pulmonary artery	13 ± 1	13 ± 1
Pulmonary capillary wedge	6 ± 1	4 ± 1
Left ventricular end diastolic	8 ± 1	4 ± 1
Stroke index (ml/m²)	50 ± 5	35 ± 3
Cardiac index (L/min/m²)	3.5 ± 0.3	2.8 ± 0.2
Ejection fraction (%)	76 ± 2	72 ± 4
Volume (ml)		
End diastolic	107 ± 10	85 ± 6
End systolic	34 ± 4	32 ± 5
Stroke	76 ± 8	55 ± 5

[a] Means ± SE for 10 sedentary men
[b] Means ± SE for 7 normal subjects
(Modified from Thadani U and Parker JO: Hemodynamics at rest and during supine and sitting bicycle exercise in normal subjects. Am J Cardiol 41:52, 1978, with permission.)

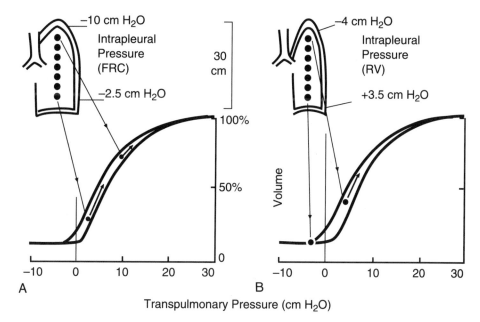

Fig. 5-1. Effect of regional differences of intrapleural pressure on the distribution of ventilation (V̇e). The pressure is assumed to fall at the rate of 0.25 cm H_2O/cm vertical distance. **(A)** At the beginning of a normal inspiration (functional residual capacity [FRC]), the transpulmonary pressures at the apex and base are assumed to be 10 and 2.5 cm H_2O, respectively. The two regions are therefore on different parts of the pressure–volume curve, and the lung units at the base have a smaller initial volume and a larger change in volume than those at the apex. V̇e therefore decreases with distance up the lung. **(B)** By contrast, at residual volume (RV), the intrapleural pressure at the base may actually exceed airway pressure so that this region is not ventilated and the airways are closed. (From West,[9] with permission.)

Distribution of Ventilation

The effect of gravity is the primary determinant of the distribution of V̇e.[9,36,37] In the upright position, the weight of the lung is supported by the rib cage and diaphragm so that a gradient in pleural pressure (Ppl) exists, wherein Ppl becomes less negative from the apex to the base of the lung as depicted in Figure 5-1A. This gradient is greatest in the vertical lung, since the lung's height is largest in this position. This Ppl gradient results in a greater regional apex volume as compared to that of the base, which places these regions on different portions of the pressure–volume curve. As a result of this difference in regional volume (Vo) and the alinear nature of the pressure–volume curve, the lung base is more compliant and receives a greater V̇e distribution than the apex. The situation at residual volume (RV) differs from that just described at functional residual capacity (FRC). The decrease in elastic recoil of the lung at RV causes the Ppl to become more positive while maintaining the apex-to-base gradient as shown in Figure 5-1B. This moves the apex and base down the pressure–volume curve so that the apex is more compliant and receives a greater distribution of the $\dot{V}e$ than the base, which has a very low Vo and is thus prone to airway closure. This situation also occurs in healthy older individuals breathing at FRC, due to the loss of elastic recoil that occurs with aging.[38]

Changes in thoracic configuration and voluntary muscle contraction have been investigated with respect to their influence on the distribution of $\dot{V}e$. Contrary to the results of animal studies, neither voluntarily induced changes of abdominal wall configuration[39] or strapping of the thorax[40] effected a change in the distribution of Vo or $\dot{V}e$ in humans. The diaphragmatic boundary is the most deformable part of the chest wall, and changes in the distribution of Vo have been demonstrated when the compliance of the diaphragm is decreased by voluntary contraction[41,42] or increased by muscle paralysis[43] in the horizontal position. The distribution of gas inspired from FRC can be influenced by healthy, trained subjects who perform abdominal or intercostal inspirations aided by biofeedback.[44] Abdominal inspiration exaggerated the normal apex-to-base gradient in $\dot{V}e$, while intercostal inspiration increased $\dot{V}e$ to the nondependent regions and resulted in a more uniform distribution of $\dot{V}e$.

The normal distribution of $\dot{V}e$ can be influenced by other factors that present in disease states.[36,37,45] For example, differences in regional compliance and resistance can occur in diseases such as emphysema and asthma, which affect the characteristics of the alveoli and airways, respectively. An area A with greater resistance or compliance than a nearby area B requires more time to fill during inspiration (i.e., has a long time constant). If this time constant exceeds the time available for inspiration, area A is less well ventilated than area B. Thus, areas with long time constants are less well ventilated and become less compliant as breathing frequency increases. In addition, emphysema also affects gas diffusion by enlarging the terminal bronchioles, thus increasing the diffusion distance and impairing the adequacy of $\dot{V}e$ to these regions. In severe lung disease, these factors become so prevalent that significant intraregional $\dot{V}e$ inhomogeneity exists, which obscures the normal interregional $\dot{V}e$ gradient.[46]

Distribution of Perfusion

The pulmonary circulation is a low pressure circuit, and thus the distribution of $\dot{Q}$ in the lung is determined by alveolar pressure (P_A) as well as pulmonary arterial (Pa) and venous ($P\bar{v}$) pressures.[9,36] Gravity significantly influences the distribution of perfusion through its effect on the hydrostatic pressure within the vessels, creating a vertical base-to-apex gradient, while P_A remains constant. This perfusion gradient is greatest in the vertical position, where lung height is the largest. The lung field can be divided into four zones based on the relative magnitude of the three pressures that determine flow.[47,48] Zone 1 refers to the apex, where PA is greater than Pa and Pv̄, so that this is a region of no blood flow. However, under normal conditions, the Pa is sufficient to maintain some flow, which likely predominates in the corner vessels tethered open by the large Vo at the apex. Zone 2 refers to the midzone, where Pa now exceeds PA, which remains greater than Pv̄. The increase in Q̇ in this zone occurs via recruitment of previously closed vessels, due to an increase in driving pressure. Zone 3 refers to the lower zone, where both Pa and Pv̄ exceed PA and Q̇ increases to its greatest degree via distension of the vessels, since Pa and Pv̄ both increase by the same magnitude down the lung. Zone 4 refers to the lung base, where there is a decrease in perfusion. Mechanisms that have been suggested to explain this zone of decreased flow include increased interstitial pressure due to dependent edema and the weight of the lung, compression of the vessels due to the low Vo in this region, and hypoxic vasoconstriction due to hypoxia secondary to airway closure.

In addition to this vertical gradient of Q̇, recent work by Hakim et al.[49,50] using single-photon emission computed tomography has demonstrated a central-to-peripheral, or radial, gradient. These investigators concluded that factors other than gravity, such as conductance of the vessels, also play an important role in the distribution of Q̇.

The normal distribution of Q̇ can be influenced by factors that alter Pa, Pv̄, PA, or the vasculature itself. A decrease in Pa due to right heart failure or a decrease in circulating volume results in the development of zone 1 in the lung.[51] An increase in Pa during exercise or left-to-right intracardiac shunts results in recruitment of the upper lung and an overall more uniform distribution of perfusion. In pulmonary vascular hypertension, Q̇ is also more evenly distributed, although flow is not generally increased. The presence of obstructive lung disease or positive pressure V̇e increases PA disproportionately to Pa, so that the presence of zone 1 in the lung becomes significant and physiologic dead space (V$_D$) increases.[52,53]

Ventilation–Perfusion Matching

The effect of upright positioning on these components of O_2 transport is best integrated by considering the effect on ventilation–perfusion (V̇$_A$:Q̇) matching. Both V̇e and Q̇ increase from the apex to the base of the upright lung. Q̇ increases to a greater extent than V̇e, however, so that the V̇$_A$:Q̇ ratio decreases from the apex to the base. As a result, the V̇$_A$:Q̇ ratio is high at the apex (V$_D$), low at the base (shunt effect), and approaches 0.8 in zone 2 of the lung.[9] The regional differences in V̇$_A$:Q̇ ratios are greatest in the upright position when compared to sidelying, supine, or prone, indicating that V̇e and Q̇ are less well matched in the upright position.[54,55] This is further substantiated by the greater alveolar–

arterial oxygen tension differences in the upright position compared to supine.[56,57]

Tissue Oxygenation

To complete the O_2 cascade, O_2 must be transported to the tissues and diffuse across the tissue capillary membrane. Tissue $\dot{Q}$ is determined by the metabolic activity of the tissues ($\dot{V}O_2$), the caliber of the capillaries, and the adequacy of the $\dot{Q}$. Through the mechanism of autoregulation, the metabolic activity of the specific tissues have a significant influence on determining $\dot{Q}$.[58] During upright positioning, complex regional adjustments, such as muscular and cutaneous vasoconstriction, occur to ensure blood flow is maintained to vital organs such as the heart and brain.[21] Transport to the mitochondria is further determined by the characteristics of the O_2 dissociation curve and diffusion across the tissue capillary membrane.[58] Diffusion at the tissue level is related to the distance between capillaries, capillary density, and the capillary–tissue O_2 tension gradient. Due to the effect of gravity in the upright posture, regions below the level of the heart will have a greater driving pressure, which promotes diffusion, than those above the heart.

From this understanding of the characteristics of O_2 transport in the upright position, one can now consider the effect of a change in posture on cardiopulmonary mechanics, the distribution of $\dot{V}e$ and $\dot{Q}$, and thus O_2 transport. The following sections first consider the effect of supine, prone, and sidelying positions on the healthy individual, and then discuss the effect of confounding variables on the normal state.

OXYGEN TRANSPORT AND SUPINE POSITIONING

Supine positioning is common in the clinical setting, where it is used for surgical and other invasive procedures. It serves as the reference position for hemodynamic measures, and facilitates the provision of basic care.[59,60] Supine positioning is most significant in critically ill people, who typically assume this position for prolonged periods despite its negative consequences on O_2 transport. Furthermore, this insult to O_2 transport compounds an already compromised cardiopulmonary system in the majority of these individuals. By considering the effect of supine positioning on the components of oxygen transport, perhaps we can implement this commonly used position more judiciously.

Pulmonary Mechanics

In the supine position, the diameter of the rib cage and abdomen is decreased anteroposteriorly and increased laterally.[61] These changes, due to the effect of gravity, are greatest in the abdomen, which is more compliant than the rib cage. The diaphragm is displaced cephalad due to the increased abdominal pressure, and together with the increase in thoracic blood volume, this displacement accounts for the decrease in FRC[20,62–64] shown in Table 5-1. This decrease predisposes the supine individual to airway closure, since the closing volume remains similar to that in sitting and thus may exceed FRC. Airway closure has been documented in healthy 65-year-old sitting individuals, and has also been observed in individuals as young as 44 years old when they were supine.[38] Thus, the degree of airway closure would be quite pronounced in a supine 65-year-old or older individual. The cephalad shift of the diaphragm places it at a mechanical advantage so that Vt is predominantly generated by diaphragm-abdominal displacement.[18,19] Compared to the upright posture, both anteroposterior and lateral excursions decrease in the rib cage and increase in the abdomen.[61] Static and dynamic lung compliance decrease in supine positioning as a consequence of increased pulmonary blood volume and airway closure.[62,64–66] The resistance within the respiratory system increases and is largely attributed to an increase in lung resistance secondary to the decreased FRC.[63,67,68] Thus, the mechanical load to breathe is increased in supine positioning, such that driving pressure increases to maintain the minute ventilation.[63]

Cardiovascular Mechanics

On assumption of the supine position from standing, there is a significant shift of blood volume from the lower extremities and abdomen into the thorax. This has an immediate and profound physiologic effect on the cardiovascular system and initiates the development of orthostatic intolerance as detailed in Chapter 8.[21,23,69–71] Representative values for hemodynamic parameters and left ventricular performance in supine and sitting positions are shown in Table 5-2, where it can be seen that the heart volume is significantly increased in the supine position. In fact, the heart volume is reported to be maximal in supine positioning, even to the extent that there is little change with the addition of a head-down tilt.[23] Although the increased venous return, or increased preload, leads to an enhanced SV, it also results in an increased afterload.[72] As the heart is dilated with the increased preload, the ventricular wall tension (afterload) increases in accordance with Laplace's law. In a state of increased afterload, the tension required of each myocardial fiber to overcome the increased wall tension and generate a given intraventricular pressure is greater than that in a normal state and results in increased stroke work.[73–75] In addition, because of the effects of ventricular interdependence, right ventricular dilatation shifts the interventricular septum and compromises the preload of the left ventricle while raising its pressure.[76] The decrease in left ventricular SV during inspiration, where there is an acute increase in right ventricular volume, has also been explained on this basis.[77] The occurrence of increased myocardial work in supine has been recognized in the research and clinical management of patients with cardiovascular disease.[32,78,79]

Distribution of Ventilation and Perfusion

In the supine position, there is a 30 percent reduction in the vertical height of the lung, resulting in a smaller intrapleural pressure gradient, which suggests that the distribution of $\dot{V}e$ would be more uniform than in the upright lung.[36,80] However, the gradient of expansion (ratio of change in Vo from FRC to change in vertical distance of the lung) is greater in supine positioning than in the upright lung.[37] Thus, although the distribution of $\dot{V}e$ increases from the nondependent to dependent regions as in the upright lung, the ratio of $\dot{V}e$ between these regions is greater.[81,82] In subjects with significant airway closure, however, the gradient becomes more uniform or reversed, since the dependent airways are closed at the onset of inspiration.[83] The incidence of this altered $\dot{V}e$ gradient is significant in supine positioning due to the large dependent lung surface area and the decrease in FRC.[38,62] Unlike in the upright lung, when supine there is also a horizontal gradient in $\dot{V}e$, wherein cephalad zones are better ventilated than caudal or paradiaphragmatic zones.[81,84,85] However, this gradient is smaller in magnitude than the vertical gradient, and is largely confined to the dependent part of the lung.[81] A decrease in expansion of the dependent caudal relative to cephalad regions has been observed.[86,87] The weight of the caudal mediastinum, abdominal hydrostatic pressure, and distortion of the dependent rib cage have been suggested as factors in determining this gradient.[37] The gradient is most pronounced when closing capacity exceeds FRC, so that airway closure is prevalent.[85] The distribution of $\dot{Q}$ in supine positioning is relatively more uniform throughout the lungs, and has been reported to follow the same gradient as the upright lung. Since the Pa and P$\bar{v}$ exceed PA (assumed to be atmospheric) in this position, it has been suggested that the entire lung is predominated by zone 3.[14] However, Prefaut and Engel[83] observed that the distribution of $\dot{Q}$ was either uniform or greater to the nondependent lung regions in subjects with airway closure. They concluded that the gravity-dependent gradient of $\dot{Q}$ is modified by hypoxic vasoconstriction due to dependent airway closure prevalent in the supine position. As opposed to the condition in the upright lung, the $\dot{V}_A:\dot{Q}$ ratio increases from the nondependent to dependent lung regions, due primarily to the change in $\dot{V}e$.[14] However, the distribution of the $\dot{V}_A:\dot{Q}$ ratio would also be influenced by the above-mentioned factors that alter the distribution of $\dot{V}e$ and $\dot{Q}$. Without considering these factors, the regional differences in the $\dot{V}_A:\dot{Q}$ ratio are smaller in all horizontal postures as compared to upright, suggesting that $\dot{V}e$ and $\dot{Q}$ are better matched.[55,88]

OXYGEN TRANSPORT AND PRONE POSITIONING

Pulmonary Mechanics

In the prone position, the diameters of the rib cage and abdomen are similar to those in the supine position, except for a decrease in the anteroposterior diameter of the abdomen. The abdominal anteroposterior excursion also decreases in comparison to that in supine positioning, but remains greater than the lateral excursion.[61] The diaphragm is displaced by the abdominal contents, which enhances its mechanical advantage so that it can oppose the increased abdominal pressure. Although the FRC is decreased compared to sitting, it remains greater than that in supine.[89] In a prone abdomen-free position, the FRC is greater than in the typical prone posture.[90] When turned from supine to prone, a 60 percent decrease in the total static compliance of the respiratory system has been observed and is related to the decreased compliance of the rib cage and diaphragm.[91]

Cardiovascular Mechanics

Little research has been done on the effect of prone and sidelying positioning on cardiovascular hemodynamics and mechanics. The studies that have been done present with conflicting results related to differences in subjects and measurement techniques. Most studies have used animal models or patients with unstable hemodynamic parameters, and have relied on indirect techniques to measure $\dot{Q}$.[34] Hemodynamic responses could be considered to be comparable in the prone and supine positions, since the fluid shift into the thorax would be similar. However, the cardiovascular mechanics may differ in prone compared to supine positioning, since the heart is located anterior of midline and would thus be more dependent in prone positioning, with a greater thoracic mass above it. Some evidence exists to support the role of compression in distinguishing cardiovascular mechanics in sidelying and supine positioning.[34,35] In prone positioning, the compressive force acts on the heart chambers more equally.

Distribution of Ventilation and Perfusion

Little work has been done on the effect of prone and sidelying positioning on the distribution of $\dot{V}e$ and $\dot{Q}$. In prone positioning, the lung undergoes a comparable decrease in vertical height to supine positioning, which may be modified by abdomen-free positioning. The expansion gradient is less than that in the upright lung, in both the prone and prone abdomen-free postures.[37] In the prone posture, $\dot{V}e$ is distributed uniformly in the vertical direction.[81] However, in the prone abdomen-free position, $\dot{V}e$ is greater in the dependent zones.[92] A cephalocaudal gradient has also been observed in the dependent zones in the prone position, although to a lesser magnitude than in the supine.[81] There is greater caudal V̇e in the prone position and cephalad V̇e in the prone abdomen-free position. The distribution of Q̇ and $\dot{V}_A:\dot{Q}$ ratios, and factors that influence this distribution, is comparable to that of supine positioning.[14,37]

OXYGEN TRANSPORT
AND SIDELYING POSITIONING

Pulmonary Mechanics

When moving from the supine to the sidelying position, the anteroposterior diameters of the rib cage and abdomen increase, while the lateral diameters decrease. There is an increase in the lateral excursions of the rib cage or abdomen, or both. The anteroposterior excursions of the rib cage increase or decrease, while those of the abdomen decrease. Thus, the diameters and tidal excursions change in opposite directions. Contrary to what one would expect, maximal tidal excursions occur in a direction against gravity in supine, prone, and sidelying positions. Mechanisms that have been postulated to explain this occurrence include differences in the distribution of respiratory muscle force, the activity or mechanical advantage of various inspiratory muscles, and local compliance in the rib cage and abdomen.[61] In sidelying position, the dependent hemidiaphragm is displaced cephalad so that its excursion is greater than that of the nondependent hemidiaphragm, enabling it to contribute to the greater V̇e of the dependent lung.[14,43] The FRC in sidelying positioning is intermediate between upright and supine, and the regional FRC is greater in the nondependent lung.[14,62] Intermediate values between those for sitting and supine positions have also been observed for lung compliance and resistance in sidelying position.[63,64] The decreased compliance and increased resistance and abdominal pressure increase the work of breathing (WOB) in sidelying compared to the upright position. However, a compensatory increase in driving pressure was not observed, so that minute ventilation was lower than that in sitting or supine. One mechanism suggested to explain this occurrence is that only the dependent fibers of the diaphragm are stretched by cephalad displacement, so that fewer fibers are at a mechanical advantage.[63] In addition, the anteroposterior displacement of the abdomen in sidelying position may decrease the base on which the diaphragm acts to expand the rib cage, thus decreasing its efficacy.

Cardiovascular Mechanics

Although there is limited data on the effect of the sidelying position on cardiovascular mechanics, Lange et al.[34] have obtained data using the thermodilution technique, which is highly reliable and reproducible for measuring Q̇ and its components. Specifically, they measured Q̇ in 24 hemodynamically stable patients undergoing elective cardiac catheterization. They observed that SV, HR, and Q̇ were comparable in supine, left, and right sidelying positioning. They also observed that right and left ventricular pressures increased when subjects assumed a sidelying position, as was previously demonstrated by Nakao et al.[35] in dogs and pigs. Further, Lange et al.[34] measured left ventricular end-diastolic pressure (LVEDP) and volume in supine and left sidelying positions and were able to demonstrate that the increased LVEDP in left sidelying position was due to a position-induced reduction in left ventricular compliance. They suggested that the right ventricle, pericardium, extracardiac intrathoracic structures, and high intra-abdominal organs could act to compress the left ventricle in left sidelying position. In addition, they hypothesized that the increased right ventricular pressures seen in sidelying position were also due to the same mechanism.

Distribution of Ventilation and Perfusion

In sidelying, the expansion gradient is the greatest for any of the positions.[37] The Vo gradient decreases from the upper to the lower lung and the vertical $\dot{V}e$ gradient increases.[14] The cephalocaudal gradient is intermediate in magnitude between supine and prone positioning, and predominates in the dependent lung.[81,93] $\dot{Q}$ increases from the nondependent to dependent regions of the lungs at a greater magnitude than in supine or prone positioning. Kaneko et al.[14] suggested that the upper one-third of each lung is in zone 2, while the lower two-thirds are in zone 3. These investigators reported that the $\dot{V}_A:\dot{Q}$ ratios were lowest at a point 20 cm from the dependent aspect of the lower lung and increased both above and below this point, regardless of whether the subject was in left or right sidelying position. There was an overall decrease in the ratio from the nondependent region of the upper lung to the dependent region of the lower lung.

EFFECT OF CONFOUNDING FACTORS ON OXYGEN TRANSPORT AND BODY POSITIONING

The preceding discussion of the components of O_2 transport and the influence of body positioning on these components provides a physiologic basis for determining the positioning management of a patient. On closer examination, however, the challenge of this task becomes clearer, since a specific position may optimize one aspect of O_2 transport, yet have little effect or a detrimental effect on other aspects. For instance, placing a sedated individual breathing at low lung volumes in left sidelying position would optimize $\dot{V}e$ to the nondependent zones, while optimizing $\dot{Q}$ to the dependent zones. If this individual were a postoperative coronary artery bypass graft (CABG) patient, the increased left ventricular pressure may compromise $\dot{Q}$ and place an excessive work demand on the heart. If, in addition, this individual was mechanically ventilated and had a left pleural effusion, the effect of this position would again be modified by these factors. Thus, as well as the effect of a given position on all of the components of O_2 transport, the influence of confounding factors must also be integrated so that the net effect on O_2 transport can be determined. This section discusses the physiologic effects of some of the confounding factors on O_2 transport, namely obesity, pleural effusions, mechanical $\dot{V}e$, and anesthesia, to enhance awareness of their significance and that of many other factors in treatment planning.

Obesity

The effect of obesity on O_2 transport has been studied in some detail.[94-98] In obesity, the closing volume becomes a greater proportion of FRC and contributes to the impaired $\dot{V}e$ in the dependent zones and thus the reversal of the normal apex-to-base gradient.[95,97] Although the increased thoracic mass results in an increased WOB, the O_2 cost of breathing is disproportionate to this increased load, suggesting that the respiratory muscles are also less efficient.[94,96] Thus $\dot{Q}$ is increased in obesity as the cardiac reserve is used to compensate for the increased preload and O_2 cost of breathing.[98]

Pleural Effusions

The effect of pleural effusions on gas exchange in different body positions has been studied in individuals without pulmonary disease.[99,100] The lowest PaO_2 and SaO_2 values were obtained when the individual was positioned on the affected side. However, the drop in SaO_2 that occurred was not considered clinically significant in individuals with an otherwise normal SaO_2.[99] Since an effusion decreases the magnitude of the Ppl and impairs the $\dot{V}e$ of the affected region, the results of these studies were attributed to the effect of increasing $\dot{Q}$ to a poorly ventilated region. However, if the effusion is large, $\dot{Q}$ will also be impaired, so that there is less $\dot{V}_A:\dot{Q}$ mismatch when the individual lies on the affected side, and oxygenation appears to be less position dependent.[100] The effect of unilateral lung disease on gas exchange in different body positions can be compared to that of effusions. In patients with unilateral lung disease (e.g., pneumonia or atelectasis) or postthoracotomy, oxygenation has been proven greatest when the individual is positioned with the affected side uppermost.[101-103] The decrease in oxygenation that occurred when the individuals were positioned on the affected side was also related to an increased $\dot{V}_A:\dot{Q}$ mismatch or shunt, because $\dot{Q}$ was increased to the poorly or nonventilated dependent regions.[104]

Mechanical Ventilation and Anesthesia

The effect of mechanical $\dot{V}e$ and anesthesia on O_2 transport is well documented, and the reader is urged to consult the literature for a comprehensive review.[43,105-108] Mechanical $\dot{V}e$ alters the normal distribution of $\dot{V}e$ and $\dot{Q}$, and also affects cardiovascular hemodynamics and mechanics. Mechanical $\dot{V}e$ implements a positive intrathoracic pressure and distributes the gases primarily along a path of least resistance. Thus, nondependent regions with large regional volumes at FRC will receive a greater proportion of $\dot{V}e$ than dependent zones subtended by small airways. High frequency $\dot{V}e$ is largely based on molecular diffusion, and thus its distribution is related to the diffusive characteristics of the respiratory zone.[107] The accompanying increased intrathoracic pressure impairs venous return and is considered the major contributor to the decrease in $\dot{Q}$ that has been observed. The resulting increase in extracardiac pressure exerts a complex effect on heart–lung and interventricular interaction that can be significant in the individual with underlying cardiovascular compromise.[106] The addition of anesthesia and paralysis in this population results in the lungs and thorax being expanded passively.[37] Froese and Bryan[43] observed that there was a cephalad shift of the end-expiratory position of the diaphragm when their supine or sidelying subjects were anesthetized and mechanically ventilated, or paralyzed. This shift was greatest in the dependent region of the diaphragm due to the significant abdominal pressure in this region. The dependent aspect of the diaphragm had the greatest tidal excursion in both the awake or anesthetized spontaneous breathing states. However, with the addition of muscle paralysis, this pattern was reversed, such that the greatest excursion occurred in the nondependent region, where there was little opposition by the abdominal contents. In addition, expansion of the dependent lung is further impeded by the weight of the mediastinum, the resistance of the surgical table, the increased $\dot{Q}$, and the development of interstitial edema.[109] Thus, these changes in the position and excursion of the diaphragm decrease the Vo and $\dot{V}e$ of the dependent zones while the individual is under the influence of anesthesia and muscle paralysis.

Although this discussion has focused on some of the common factors that influence the effect of body positioning on O_2 transport, it has not addressed many other factors. Factors such as the specific cardiopulmonary or multisystem pathology, alterations in the thoracic cage due to fractures or neurologic pathology, and the influence of invasive procedures (such as dialysis) have to be considered in similar detail so that their influence on O_2 transport can be integrated into treatment planning.

SUMMARY

The integration of the cardiovascular and pulmonary systems into a functional unit is essential for the transport of O_2 from the atmosphere to the metabolically active cells, and a simultaneous removal of CO_2 from the body back to the atmosphere. This chapter has focused on the optimization of each step of O_2 transport as the ultimate goal of therapeutic positioning. Thus, a foundation of the underlying physiologic mechanisms determining O_2 transport in the upright lung was established, and the influence of position as a therapeutic intervention was then considered. However, the reality is that several confounding factors also intervene to alter the effect of a specific position on a specific individual at any given point in time. The implications for practice are then threefold: (1) the relative importance of all these physiologic factors has to be assessed; (2) determining the therapeutic intervention from this assessment demands a highly integrative and physiologic problem-solving approach; and (3) the need for continuous monitoring of tissue oxygenation, the endpoint of the O_2 cascade, is essential. By approaching therapeutic positioning in this judicious manner, optimal treatment outcomes are more likely, and the long interval between patient visits can become an integrated part of the overall treatment plan.

REFERENCES

1. Ciesla N: Postural drainage, positioning, and breathing exercises. p. 56. In Mackenzie CF, Ciesla N, Imle PC, Klemic N (eds): Chest Physiotherapy in the Intensive Care Unit. Williams and Wilkins, Baltimore, MD, 1981
2. Frownfelter DL: Postural drainage. p. 271. In Frownfelter DL (ed): Chest Physical Therapy and Pulmonary Rehabilitation. Year Book Medical Publishers, Chicago, 1987
3. Gaskell DV, Webber BA: The Brompton Hospital Guide to Chest Physiotherapy. p. 13. 4th Ed. Blackwell Scientific Publications, Oxford, 1980
4. Haas A, Pinedo H, Haas F et al: p. 123. Pulmonary Therapy and Rehabilitation Principles and Practice. Williams and Wilkins, Baltimore, 1979
5. Reinisch ES: Functional approach to chest physical therapy: clinical Report. Phys Ther 58:972, 1978
6. Dantzker DR: Oxygen transport and utilization. Respir Care 33:874, 1988
7. Dean E: Effect of body position on pulmonary function. Phys Ther 65:613, 1985
8. Ross J, Dean E: Integrating physiological principles into the comprehensive management of cardiopulmonary dysfunction. Phys Ther 69:255, 1989
9. West JB: p. 1. Ventilation/Blood Flow and Gas Exchange. 4th Ed. Blackwell Scientific Publications, Oxford, 1985
10. Dantzker DR: The influence of cardiovascular function on gas exchange. Clin Chest Med 4:149, 1983
11. Johnson Jr RL: Heart–lung interactions in the transport of oxygen. p. 5. In Scharf SM and Cassidy SS (eds): Heart-Lung Interactions in Health and Disease. Mercel Dekker, New York, 1989
12. Weber KT, Janicki JS, Shroff SG et al: The cardiopulmonary unit. The body's gas transport system. Clin Chest Med 4:101, 1983
13. Ferris BG: Epidemiology standardization procedures for pulmonary function testing (part 2). Am Rev Respir Dis 118:55, 1978
14. Kaneko K, Milic-Emili J, Dolovich MB et al: Regional distribution of ventilation and perfusion as a function of body position. J Appl Physiol 21:767, 1966
15. Druz WS, Sharp JT: Activity of respiratory muscles in upright and recumbent humans. J Appl Physiol 51:1552, 1981
16. Druz WS, Sharp JT: Electrical and mechanical activity of the diaphragm accompanying body position in severe chronic obstructive pulmonary disease. Am Rev Respir Dis 125:275, 1982
17. Mead J: Responses to loaded breathing: a critique and a synthesis. Bull Physiopathol Respir 15:61, 1979
18. De Troyer A: Mechanical role of the abdominal muscles in relation to posture. Respir Physiol 53:341, 1983

19. Sharp JT, Goldberg NB, Druz WS et al: Relative contributions of rib cage and abdomen to breathing in normal subjects. J Appl Physiol 39:608, 1975
20. Svanberg L: Influence of posture on the lung volumes, ventilation and circulation of normals. Scand J Clin Lab Invest 25:1, 1957
21. Blomqvist CG, Stone HL: Cardiovascular adjustments to gravitational stress. p. 1,025. In Shepherd JT, Abboud FM (eds): Handbook of Physiology. American Physiological Society, Bethesda, MD, 1983
22. Rowell LB: Human Circulation Regulation During Physical Stress. p. 137. Oxford University Press, New York, 1986
23. Gauer OH, Thron HL: Postural changes in the circulation. p. 2,409. In Hamilton WF (ed): Handbook of Physiology. American Physiological Society, Washington, D.C. 1965
24. Rowell LB: Cardiovascular adjustments to thermal stress. p. 927. In Shepherd JT, Abboud FM, Geiger SR (eds): Handbook of Physiology. American Physiological Society, Bethesda, MD, 1983
25. Sjostrand T: The regulation of the blood distribution in man. Acta Physiol Scand 26:312, 1952
26. Bevegard S, Lodin A: Postural circulatory changes at rest and during exercise in five patients with congenital absence of valves in the deep veins of the legs. Acta Med Scand 172:21, 1962
27. Stegall HF: Muscle pumping in the dependent leg. Circ Res 19:180, 1966
28. Amberson WR: Physiologic adjustments to the standing posture. Bull Maryland Univ Sch Med 27:127, 1943
29. Wang Y, Marshall RJ, Shepherd JT: The effect of changes in posture and of graded exercise on stroke volume in man. J Clin Invest 39:1051, 1960
30. Moreno AH, Burchell AR, van der Woude R et al: Respiratory regulation of splanchnic and venous return. Am J Physiol 213:455, 1967
31. Marshall RJ, Shepherd JT: Cardiac Function in Health and Disease. WB Saunders, Philadelphia, 1968
32. Langou RA, Wolfson S, Olson EG, et al: Effects of orthostatic postural changes on myocardial oxygen demands. Am J Cardiol 39:418, 1977
33. Prakash R, Parmley WW, Dikshit K et al: Hemodynamic effects of postural changes in patients with acute myocardial infarction. Chest 64:7, 1973
34. Lange RA, Katz J, McBride W et al: Effects of supine and lateral positions on cardiac output and intracardiac pressures. Am J Cardiol 62:330, 1988
35. Nakao S, Come PC, Miller MJ et al: Effects of supine and lateral positions on cardiac output and intracardiac pressures: an experimental study. Circulation 73:579, 1986
36. Bates DV: Respiratory Function in Disease. 3rd Ed. WB Saunders, Philadelphia, 1989
37. Hughes JMB, Amis TC: Regional ventilation distribution. p. 177. In Engel LA, Paiva M (eds): Gas Mixing and Distribution in the Lung. Marcel Dekker, New York, 1985
38. Leblanc P, Ruff F, Milic-Emili J: Effects of age and body position on airway closure in man. J Appl Physiol 28:448, 1970
39. Grassino AE, Bake B, Martin RR et al: Voluntary changes of thoracoabdominal shape and regional lung volumes in humans. J Appl Physiol 39:997, 1975
40. Sybrecht GW, Garrett L, Anthonisen NR: Effect of chest strapping on regional lung function. J Appl Physiol 39:707, 1975
41. Roussos CH, Fukuchi Y, Macklem PT et al: Influence of diaphragmatic contraction on ventilation distribution in horizontal man. J Appl Physiol 40:417, 1976

42. Roussos CH, Martin RR, Engel LA: Diaphragmatic contraction and the gradient of alveolar expansion in the lateral posture. J Appl Physiol 43:32, 1977b

43. Froese AB, Bryan AC: Effects of anesthesia and paralysis on diaphragmatic mechanics in man. Anesthesiology 41:242, 1974

44. Roussos CH, Fixley M, Genest J et al: Voluntary factors influencing the distribution of inspired gas. Am Rev Respir Dis 116:457, 1977a

45. Milic-Emili J: Ventilation. p. 167. In West JB (ed): Regional Differences in the Lung. Academic Press, San Diego, 1977

46. Andersen LH, Rasmussen FV: Underestimation of closing volume with increase in airflow obstruction. Clin Respir Physiol 17:823, 1981

47. West JB, Dollery CT: Distribution of blood flow and the pressure–flow relations of the whole lung. J Appl Physiol 20:175, 1965

48. Hughes JMB, Glazier JB, Maloney JE et al: Effect of lung volume on the distribution of pulmonary blood flow in man. Respir Physiol 4:58, 1968

49. Hakim TS, Lisbona R, Dean GW: Gravity-independent inequality in pulmonary blood flow in humans. J Appl Physiol 63:1,114, 1987

50. Hakim TS, Lisbona R, Dean GW: Effect of body posture on spatial distribution of pulmonary blood flow. J Appl Physiol 64:1,160, 1988

51. Naimark A, Dugard A, Rangno RE: Regional pulmonary blood flow and gas exchange in hemorrhagic shock. J Appl Physiol 25:301, 1968

52. Bindslev LG, Hedenstierna G, Santesson J et al: Ventilation–perfusion distribution during inhalation anaesthesia. Acta Anaesthesiol Scand 25:360, 1981

53. Dantzker DR, Brook CJ, DeHart P et al: Ventilation–perfusion distributions in the adult respiratory distress syndrome. Am Rev Respir Dis 120:1,039, 1979

54. Bryan AC, Bentivoglio LG, Beerel F et al: Factors affecting regional distribution of ventilation and perfusion in the lung. J Appl Physiol 19:395, 1964

55. West JB, Dollery CT: Distribution of blood flow and ventilation–perfusion ratio in the lung, measured with radioactive carbon dioxide. J Appl Physiol 15:405, 1960

56. Martin CJ, Cline Jr F, Marshall H: Lobar alveolar gas concentrations. Effect of body position. J Clin Invest 32:617, 1953

57. Riley RL, Permutt S, Said S et al: Effect of posture on pulmonary dead space in man. J Appl Physiol 14:339, 1959

58. Berne RM, Levy MN: Cardiovascular Physiology. 4th Ed. CV Mosby, St. Louis, MO, 1981

59. Brown Jr RB, Blitt CD, Vaughan RW: Positioning and observation of the patient during the surgical period. p. 215. In Burnell RB, Blitt CD (eds): Clinical Anesthesiology, CV Mosby, St. Louis, MO, 1985

60. Swan HJC: Techniques of monitoring seriously ill patients with heart disease and computer-based monitoring after cardiac surgery. p. 1,998. In Hurst JW (ed): The Heart. 6th Ed. McGraw-Hill, New York, 1986

61. Vellody VP, Nassery M, Druz WS, Sharp JT: Effects of body position change on thoracoabdominal motion. J Appl Physiol 45:581, 1978

62. Agostoni E, Mead J: Statics of the respiratory system. In Fenn WO, Rahn H (eds): Handbook of Physiology. American Physiological Society, Washington, D.C. 1965

63. Baydur A, Behrakis PK, Zin WA et al: Effect of posture on ventilation and breathing pattern during room air breathing at rest. Lung 165:341, 1987

64. Behrakis PK, Baydur A, Jaeger MJ, Milic-Emili J: Lung mechanics in sitting and horizontal body positions. Chest 83:643, 1983

65. Sasaki H, Hida W, Takishima T: Influence of body position on dynamic compliance in young subjects. J Appl Physiol 42:706, 1977

66. Sutherland PW, Katsura T, Milic-Emili J: Previous volume history of the lung and regional distribution of gas. J Appl Physiol 25:566, 1968

67. Navajas D, Farre R, Rotger MM et al: Effect of body posture on respiratory impedance. J Appl Physiol 64:194, 1988

68. Sharp JT, Henry JP, Sweany SK et al: The total work of breathing in normal and obese men. J Clin Invest 43:728, 1964

69. Chobanian AV, Lille RD, Tercyak A: The metabolic and hemodynamic effects of prolonged bed rest in normal subjects. Circulation 49:551, 1974

70. Hahn-Winslow E: Cardiovascular consequences of bed rest. Heart Lung 14:236, 1985

71. Sandler H: Cardiovascular effects of inactivity. p. 11. In Sandler H, Vernikos J (eds): Inactivity: Physiological Effects. Academic Press, Orlando, FL, 1986

72. Braunwald E: Assessment of cardiac performance. p. 409. In Braunwald E (ed): Heart Disease, A Textbook of Cardiovascular Medicine. WB Saunders, Philadelphia, 1980

73. Maughan WL, Oikawa RY: Right ventricular function. p. 179. In Scharf SM, Cassidy SS (eds): Heart-Lung Interactions in Health and Disease. Marcel Dekker, New York, 1989

74. Sonnenblick EH, Ross Jr J, Braunwald E: Oxygen consumption of the heart: newer concepts of its multifactorial determination. Am J Cardiol 22:328, 1968

75. Sunagawa K, Maughan WL, Sagawa K: Optimal arterial resistance for the maximal stroke work studied in isolated canine left ventricle. Circ Res 56:586, 1985

76. Janicki JS, Shroff SG, Weber KT: Ventricular Interdependence. p. 285. In Scharf SM and Cassidy SS (eds): Heart-Lung Interactions in Health and Disease. Marcel Dekker, New York, 1989

77. Robotham JL: Cardiovascular disturbances in chronic respiratory insufficiency. Am J Cardiol 47:941, 1981

78. Spann Jr JF, Hurst JW: Recognition and management of heart failure. p. 345. In Hurst JW (ed): The Heart. 6th Ed. McGraw-Hill Book, New York, 1986

79. Parker JO, Ledwich JR, West RO et al: Reversible cardiac failure during angina pectoris. Hemodynamic effects of atrial pacing in coronary artery disease. Circulation 39:745, 1969

80. Daly WJ, Bondurant S: Direct measurement of respiratory pleural pressure changes in normal man. J Appl Physiol 18:513, 1963

81. Amis TC, Jones HA, Hughes JMB: Effect of posture on interregional distribution of pulmonary ventilation in man. Respir Physiol 56:145, 1984

82. Valind S, Rhodes CG, Clarke J et al: Quantitative measurements of regional ventilation using positron computed tomography [PCT] and a short-lived inert gas-Neon-19. Nucl Med Commun 4:149, 1983

83. Prefaut CH, Engel LA: Vertical distribution of perfusion and inspired gas in supine man. Respir Physiol 43:209, 1981

84. Bynum LJ, Wilson JE, Pierce AK: Comparison of spontaneous and positive pressure breathing in supine normal subjects. J Appl Physiol 41:341, 1976

85. Engel LA, Prefaut CH: Cranio-caudal distribution of inspired gas and perfusion in supine man. Respir Physiol 45:43–53, 1981

86. Bake B, Bjure J, Grimby E et al: Regional distribution of inspired gas in supine man. Scand J Respir Dis 48:189, 1967

87. Sybrecht G, Landau L, Murphy BG et al: Influence of posture on flow dependence of distribution of inhaled 133Xe boli. J Appl Physiol 41:489, 1976

88. Anthonisen NR, Milic-Emili J: Distribution of pulmonary perfusion in erect man. J Appl Physiol 21:760, 1966

89. Agostoni E, Hyatt RE: Static behavior of the respiratory system (part 1). p. 113. In Macklem PT, Mead J (eds): Handbook of Physiology. American Physiological Society, Bethesda, MD, 1986

90. Douglas WW, Rehder K, Beynen FM et al: Improved oxygenation in patients with acute respiratory failure: the prone position. Am Rev Respir Dis 115:559, 1977

91. Lynch S, Brand, L Levy A: Changes in lung thoracic compliance during orthopedic surgery. Anesthesiology 20:278, 1959

92. Rehder K, Knopp TJ, Sessler AD: Regional intrapulmonary gas distribution in awake and anesthetized paralyzed prone man. J Appl Physiol 45:528, 1978

93. Demedts M: Regional distribution of lung volumes, ventilation and transpulmonary pressures. Thesis, Departement Pathofysiologie, Facultiet der Geneeskunde, Katholieke Universiteit Leuven, Leuven, Belgium, 1978

94. Cherniack RM, Guenter CA: The efficiency of the respiratory muscles in obesity. J Biochem Physiol Can 39:1,215, 1961

95. Don HF, Craig DB, Wahba WM et al: The measurement of gas trapped in the lungs at functional residual capacity and the effect of posture. Anesthesiology 35:582, 1971

96. Fritts Jr WW, Filler J, Fishman AP et al: The efficiency of ventilation during voluntary hyperpnea: studies in normal subjects and in dyspneic patients with either chronic pulmonary emphysema or obesity. J Clin Invest 38:1,339, 1959

97. Hurewitz AN, Susskind H, Harold WH: Obesity alters regional ventilation in lateral decubitus position. J Appl Physiol 59:774, 1985

98. Paul DR, Hoyt JL, Boutros AR: Cardiovascular and respiratory changes in response to change of posture in the very obese. Anesthesiology 45:73, 1976

99. Neagley SR, Zwillich CW: The effect of positional changes on oxygenation in patients with pleural effusions. Chest 88:714, 1985

100. Sonnenblick M, Melzer E, Rosin AJ: Body positional effect on gas exchange in unilateral pleural effusion. Chest 83:784, 1983

101. Remolina C, Khan AU, Santiago TV, et al: Positional hypoxemia in unilateral lung disease. N Engl J Med 304:523, 1981

102. Seaton D, Lapp NL, Morgan WKC: Effect of body position on gas exchange after thoracotomy. Thorax 34:518, 1979

103. Zach MB, Pontoppidan H, Kazemi H: The effect of lateral positions on gas exchange in pulmonary disease. Am Rev Respir Dis 110:49, 1974

104. Fishman AP: Down with the good lung (editorial). N Engl J Med 304:537, 1981

105. Covino BG, Fozzard HA, Rehder K, Strichartz G (eds): Effects of Anesthesia. p. 75. American Physiological Society, Bethesda, MD, 1985

106. Dhainaut JF, Aouate P, Brunet FP: Circulatory effects of positive end-expiratory pressure in patients with acute lung injury. p. 809. In Scharf SM, Cassidy SS (eds): Heart-Lung Interactions in Health and Disease. Marcel Dekker, New York, 1989

107. Slutsky AS, Kamm RD, Drazen JM: Alveolar ventilation at high frequencies using tidal volumes smaller than the anatomical dead space. p. 137. In Scharf SM, Cassidy SS (eds): Heart-Lung Interactions in Health and Disease. Marcel Dekker, New York, 1989

108. Vincent JL, Suter PM: Cardiopulmonary Interactions in Acute Respiratory Failure. p. 1. Springer-Verlag, New York, 1987

109. Potgieter SV: Atelectasis: its evolution during upper urinary tract surgery. Br J Anaesth 31:472, 1959

6 | Manual Techniques of Chest Physical Therapy and Airway Clearance Techniques

Julie A. Starr

In the healthy respiratory system, the goblet cells of the tracheobronchial tree produce a thin layer of mucus (less than 5 μm) that is continually swept upstream toward the glottis, maintaining a clear and patent airway.[1] Certain pulmonary diseases cause abnormalities in this normal cleansing process through (1) an increase in the production of the goblet cells, (2) a change in the biochemical and physical properties of the goblet cell secretions, or (3) an alteration in the action of the cilia within the tracheobronchial tree.[2] When the mucus overwhelms the functioning of the mucociliary transport system, gas exchange is hampered.

The manual techniques of chest physical therapy, namely percussion, shaking, vibration, and airway clearance maneuvers, such as coughing and suctioning, are empirically used to remove retained secretions from the tracheobronchial tree, thereby promoting more effective aeration throughout the lungs. The specific action of these techniques has not been rigorously or completely studied, but attempts have been made to measure their effectiveness.[3] The literature encompassing the chest physical therapy manual techniques seems fraught with inconsistencies and contradictions, making a definitive and systematic evaluation of these techniques somewhat difficult. Initially, this chapter briefly discusses the difficulties encountered when interpreting the current research on chest physical therapy manual techniques. The performance of each manual technique and each airway clearance maneuver is then described, and through literature review, what is known and what needs to be known about its action and effectiveness is discussed.

INCONSISTENCIES WITHIN THE LITERATURE

To critically review the manual techniques of chest physical therapy, we must acknowledge inconsistencies in nomenclature of manual techniques. *Percussion* is a technique that also has been referred to as tapotement,[4] pummelling,[5] cupping,[6] and clapping.[7,8] The terms *shaking* and *vibration* are sometimes used interchangeably by clinicians, educators, and researchers. In other instances, they refer to two different techniques: shaking, which provides chest wall compression and displacement, and vibration, which does not. The terms *postural drainage* and *bronchial drainage* have been used to refer both to certain body positions that employ gravity to enhance secretion clearance from the lung segments,[9] and to an entire treatment program consisting of manual chest percussion, vibration, and cough instruction, along with these body positions.[10,11]

Comparing research results is also difficult when one study uses a single technique as an independent variable[7,12] (i.e., percussion), and another study uses a combination of techniques[8,10] (i.e., percussion with shaking and coughing in a postural drainage position). The evaluation of a single manual technique may be methodologically sound, but the clinical significance of such a study is difficult to ascertain. Zidulka et al.[7] evaluated lateral chest wall percussion on anaethetized dogs in the supine position. Percussion performed for 10 minutes was found to cause atelectasis by postmortem study. However, percussion is rarely performed as a single technique. Some method of postural drainage, shaking and cough, or suctioning usually accompanies the technique. Could there be compound effects of these techniques? The clinical significance of percussions's efficacy within a treatment program remains unanswered.

Chest physical therapy manual techniques are clinically performed in combination, yet studying them this way has confounding results. Lorin and Denning compared a treatment program consisting of postural drainage, percussion, shaking, and directed coughing to spontaneous coughing in the sitting position, to find that the treatment group produced more than twice the sputum that the control group did.[10] Using therapeutic regimens as they are clinically performed during research studies does not address such issues as (1) which part of the treatment program is most effective, (2) what possible cumulative effects do these techniques have, and (3) is it necessary to include all techniques to achieve the same results.

A third source of variation among study findings is the broad application of these techniques to a diagnostically diverse population. Some researchers use subjects with healthy respiratory systems,[13] while others study respiratory systems with active disease processes.[14,15] Another population often studied is postoperative patients.[5,16,17] These groups of healthy, diseased, and postsurgical subjects range from animals[12] to humans[18–20] and neonates[21,22] to adults.[23,24]

With such a spectrum of subjects being referenced, comparison of research findings on the manual techniques is questionable.

The effectiveness measurements used in evaluating the manual techniques also can lead to intrastudy discrepencies. Measured outcomes of chest physical therapy techniques have included the volume of secretions raised,[8,11,16,25] pulmonary function test results,[6,11,26,27] oxygenation,[22,23,28–31] chest radiograph interpretation,[32] participants' subjective impression,[24] radioactive tagged particle clearance,[12,33–35] thoracic–lung compliance,[36] length of hospital stay,[20] development of postoperative pulmonary complications,[5,37] and exercise performance.[38] When we review research conclusions with such varied evaluation endpoints, generalizations become intuitive at best.

The lack of standardization in the performance of each technique is a fifth source for variation among research.[8,21,39] Percussion is rarely qualified by its frequency, intensity, duration, or location. A clinician or mechanical device may be performing the technique. The same lack of qualifiers exists for shaking and vibration.

A final variation in the literature surrounding the effectiveness of chest physical therapy techniques is the time elapsed between technique application and outcome measurement. Does the effect of the manual techniques extend beyond the time it takes to perform them? Evaluation endpoints have been measured immediately following the therapy session,[2,7] 1 to 2 hours posttherapy (short-term effect),[25,40] and 3 years later (long-term effect).[41] The question of how long following the completion of the therapy session effects should be measured remains unanswered.

The following sections review the present literature on the evaluation of the manual techniques (percussion, shaking, and vibration) and airway clearance (cough, cough variants, and suctioning) with the above-mentioned problems in mind. This chapter defines what we do, what we know, as well as what we should know about these therapeutic measures.

MANUAL TECHNIQUES OF CHEST PHYSICAL THERAPY

Percussion

What We Do

Chest percussion is generally defined as a downward force rhythmically applied by the physical therapist's cupped hands to the patients thorax over the involved lung segment(s). Inductively, percussing the thorax creates an energy wave that is transmitted through the chest wall to the underlying lung tissue.[42] Vibrations are caused within the generations of bronchi in that area, enhancing secretion clearance from that lung segment. Adapted equipment, such as padded medicine cups, anesthesia masks, and mechanical percussors, are sometimes used to perform percussion, to achieve the same results. Zadai[43] documented that in 1934, Linton observed the percussion technique to "splatter" the secretions from the wall of the tracheobronchial tree.

Indication for percussion is excessive sputum production or retention. Percussion is usually preceded by the appropriate postural drainage position and followed by shaking or vibration to increase the probability of secretion removal.

Since percussion is a force directed to the thorax, many clinicians have cited relative contraindications to be considered prior to its use.[9,44–46] Many of the conditions discussed below are presented to make the user aware of possible untoward events; however, the clinical literature continually dispells objections to the use of a given manual technique.[6,47–49] These conditions, therefore, are not intended to discourage the use of percussion, but to encourage the making of an appropriate decision after weighing benefits against possible detriments, on an individual patient basis.

Precautions

Dysfunctional Circulatory System. A dysfunctional circulatory system may require the therapist to closely monitor patient tolerance to a treatment program that includes the percussion technique. In the recent past, a precordial thump had been used in cardiopulmonary resuscitation to cardiovert an arrhythmia into normal sinus rhythm. It has been postulated that unsteady cardiac rhythms might be subject to negative changes with the use of percussion. Simple monitoring of the electrocardiogram during percussion can uncover any arrhythmias.

Coagulation Disorders. The benefits of percussion in patients with coagulation disorders should be carefully weighed against possible complications. Some authors encourage caution prior to the use of percussion when encountering a patient with an increased partial thromboplastin time (PTT) or prothrombin time (PT), a decreased platelet count, or the use of thrombolytic drugs such as tissue-type plasminogen activator (tPA), streptokinase or urokinase.[44] However, other institutions vary the vigor with which the technique is performed, based on the underlying pathology, rather than electing not to performed it.[50] Monitoring the thorax for bruising or petechiae is of limited value, as doing so does not warn of any impending untoward effect, but rather only informs that one has occurred.

Frank Hemoptysis. This should be documented and assessed. Whether this contraindicates the use of percussion should be weighed against how the patient will clear the airways without the manual technique. Certainly, repetitive unassisted coughing in a patient with retained secretions is contraindicated when hemoptysis is present. The use of percussion and shaking in a postural drainage position, along with a version of the cough maneuver that lowers the transpulmonary pressure[51] (i.e., huff[52] a cough without a closed glottis) or forced expiration technique[53,54]([FET] an expiratory manuever performed from lower lung volumes in conjunction with controlled breathing), may be less likely to increase the amount of bleeding within the pulmonary system than frequent coughing at high intrathoracic pressures that may occur with the abandonment of the manual techniques. A case study of fatal pulmonary hemorrhage in a patient who had a squamous cell carcinoma and a lung abscess was reported by Hammon and Martin[55] in 1979. After 16 days of physical therapy, the patient died of pulmonary hemorrhage. The conclusion was that percussion caused the exsanguination of the patient. Kigin rebuked these conclusions, stating that hemoptysis is a known complication for carcinoma, for pulmonary abscess, and for coughing.[3] The patient was admitted with hemoptysis and continued to have hemoptysis during the entire course of his hospital admission. Therefore, the conclusion that percussion was the cause seems somewhat presumptuous.

Rib Fractures and Flail Chests. Percussion has been avoided in some patients with fractured ribs and flail chests because of the possibility of causing an extrapulmonary hematoma or a pneumothorax. In a 1987 study by Ciesla et al.,[47] there were no apparent sequelae to the use of percussion in 250 patients with multiple rib fractures. A word of caution needs to be given, however, as most of the patients in this series were on controlled mechanical ventilation during the physical therapy treatment. The authors suggested that controlled positive pressure ventilation acts as a splint to keep the rib fractures fixed. Percussion in this population may have caused less rib motion than in a population employing spontaneous breathing, coughing, or even assisted or intermittent mandatory ventilation.

Degenerative Bone Disease. The use of percussion has been questioned in patients with degenerative bone disease. There is obviously no desire to cause the pain and dysfunction that accompany a rib fracture. However, patients can fracture ribs with coughing alone. Again, questions arise: what course of treatment is less detrimental to the patient? Could the combination of postural drainage, percussion, and vibration, along with external splinting and a huff or an FET—used to move secretions centrally—be less detrimental than unassisted high intrathoracic pressures produced by repetative vigorous coughing alone?

Intracranial Pressure. Intracranial pressure had been thought to increase during percussion, postural drainage, and shaking, and therefore was considered a contraindication to the use of percussion. Raval et al.[56] reported that a group of neonates receiving chest physical therapy and suctioning had a higher incidence of intraventricular hemorrhage than did a control group receiving suctioning alone. However, percussion alone in the adult population is not linked to an elevated intracranial pressure.[49] The use of percussion, even in conjunction with postural drainage, does not significantly alter the cerebral perfusion pressure,[48] although intracranial pressure may rise.[57]

Pain. Pain may contraindicate the use of percussion. However, there are many aspects to pain that should be evaluated before rejecting percussion as an appropriate treatment technique. Pain such as that with pleuritis will not be made worse by the use of manual techniques; therefore, this type of pain does not contraindicate percussion. A respiratory dysfunction caused by pain, such as that with a postoperative incision, may be made worse by the use of percussion. However, in the postoperative patient, everything is painful—deep breathing, turning, coughing, walking, laughing, and so forth. Careful administration of analgesics, proper positioning, and the use of proper splinting prior to the use of the manual techniques are appropriate pain-prevention measures. Imle[50] holds the following interesting view: since the avoidance of percussion will not lessen the pain, percussion with appropriate analgesia should be used if necessary.

Increased bronchospasm. Campbell et al.[27] and Wollmer et al.[19] documented a decrease in forced expiratory volume in one second (FEV_1) with the use of percussion in patients with chronic bronchitis. Many researchers do not correlate a decrease in expiratory flow measures with the use of percussion.[6,26,58,59] Huber et al.[6] found a 40 percent improvement in FEV_1 after the use of percussion in asthmatic patients who were known to become bronchospastic with the treatment. Feldman et al.[26] also found improvement in FEV_1 5, 15, and 45 minutes after percussion, vibration, and coughing in postural drainage positions in their cystic fibrosis patients, though this change did not occur in their chronic bronchitic patients. Although the data seem conflicting, with the proper use of bronchodilator therapy and frequent assessment of breath sounds during treatment, percussion can be instituted with bronchospastic patients.

What We Know

Patient populations with widely differing diagnoses are used in the current research. Below is a description of some of the populations studied and the results specific to those sampled.

Percussion has been shown to be beneficial in the removal of chronic excessive secretions from the tracheobronchial tree. Bateman et al.[33] showed that in adult patients whose secretion production was 100 ml/24 hours, percussion increased the amount of secretions expectorated. Cochrane et al.[25] and Mazzocco et al.[15] have also found percussion to increase the amount of secretions expectorated in chronically overproductive adult patients. Denton[8] and Etches and Scott[60] have shown that percussion increases the amount of secretions expectorated in pediatric patients.

Percussion does not assist in secretion clearance in patients who have chronically minimal secretions. Campbell et al.[27] and Newton and Stevenson[61] evaluated percussion in their adult chronic bronchitic patients whose reported sputum production was between 5 and 30 ml/day. Physical therapy manuevers in this patient population did not improve secretion removal.

Mackenzie[62] found that even though acutely ill patients may have minimal secretion expectoration, percussion has a positive benefit. The specific area of clearance, rather than the amount of secretions cleared, has been credited with improved pulmonary function.

Percussion has actually been shown to be detrimental in subjects with no apparent pulmonary disorders. Zidluka et al.[7] showed that in anesthetized artificially ventilated healthy mongrel dogs, atelectasis could be induced with 10 minutes of percussion. Reines[5] looked at children after cardiac surgery without any defined pulmonary dysfunction and showed that the institution of percussion, along with positioning caused an increase in the occurrence of postoperative atelectasis.

In summary, the populations studied have demonstrated that there must be a pulmonary dysfunction amenable to the techniques used to achieve ventilation improvement. Since the indication for percussion is excessive secretions, then patients most likely to benefit from it would have excessive secretions. In the now famous analogy by Murray,[63] the ketchup bottle must contain some ketchup before it can be emptied.

As shown in the above review, neonatal, pediatric, adult, and geriatric patients seem to benefit equally from the use of percussion. There may be a difference in the resonant frequencies of the thorax of pediatric and adult patients. Optimal frequency and intensity of percussion are addressed later in this discussion.

Effectiveness Evaluation Methods

Methods of measuring the effectiveness of percussion vary among studies. Different evaluation methods are presented and compared in the following sections.

Secretion Production.   Secretions have been measured by both volume and dry weight. Denton,[8] Mazzocco,[15] Bateman et al.,[33] and Cochrane et al.[25] all found percussion to increase the amount of sputum produced during their experimental sessions. Etches and Scott[60] observed that the weight of secretions suctioned from their neonatal subjects was significantly greater when percussion and vibration were performed than when no manual techniques were used. The opposite effect was reported by Murphy,[64] who found the addition of percussion to postural drainage actually decreased sputum production in the two cystic fibrosis patients evaluated. The methodology allowed percussion to be interrupted every 20 to 30 seconds for shaking, deep breathing, coughing, and FET.

The sole use of measured sputum production to assess the efficacy of percussion is not without flaws. Swallowed secretions, saliva produced with secretions, and the period during which secretion expectoration is measured all plague its use.

Oxygenation.   The partial pressure of arterial oxygen (PaO_2), oxygen saturation (SaO_2), and transcutaneous oxygen tension ($TcPO_2$) have been used to evaluate the efficacy of percussion. Finer and Boyd[21] reported that infants significantly improved their PaO_2 values when percussion was added to the control treatment of postural drainage. Crane et al.[22] compared percussion with vibration in two different drainage positions. $TcPO_2$ measured 30 minutes before treatment, and 5, 15, and 60 minutes after treatment, showed an upward trend that did not reach statistical significance. Tudehope and Bagley[65] demonstrated an improved PaO_2 after two types of manual percussion (one with the heel of the hand, one with a face mask) were performed on premature infants.

Raval et al.[66] found a significant decrease in $TcPO_2$ in seven infants who received percussion and vibration for 1 minute in two positions; however, endotracheal suctioning was performed without hyperinflation or hyperoxygenation prior to the measurement of $TcPO_2$. Holloway et al.[67] also noted a drop in PaO_2 with percussion and vibration with endotracheal suctioning over each lung area drained. Once hyperinflation and hyperoxygenation were instituted, no drop in PaO_2 was observed.

In summary, it appears that oxygenation can be affected by percussion. Patients who are unable to maintain adequate oxygenation during percussion may require oxygen support.

Mucociliary Transport Velocities. The movement of inhaled aerosolized particles within the tracheobronchial tree can be followed by using gamma cameras, scintillation counters, fluoroscopic units, or cinefibroscopic technique. The particle movement is an objective measure of mucociliary clearance. This methodology has been used in the current research to evaluate efficacy of manual chest physical therapy techniques on mucociliary clearance within the lungs.

Chopra et al.[12] showed that the sole use of percussion in anesthetized dogs increased the tracheal transport velocity (TTV) by 51 percent when compared to a control period of rest. The addition of percussion to a treatment session of postural drainage and coughing in three experimental animals showed a further increase in TTV, though no further statistical significance could be documented. These results were confirmed by Van der Schans et al.[68] Sutton et al.[69] incorporated percussion into a treatment session of postural drainage and voluntary coughing and documented that clearance of the radioaerosol was not significantly altered by the addition of percussion, although there was an increase in the dry weight of secretions. Rossman et al.[70] confirmed that the clearance of radioaerosolized particles during postural drainage was not significantly enhanced by the addition of percussion. However, the volumes of sputum expectorated immediately after the treatment session and 2 hours later were greatest when the treatment included percussion.

Performance of the Technique

In the earlier studies on the manual techniques, there were no clear operational definitions. Methodology stated that the techniques were performed, but there was no indication as to the intensity, frequency, or duration of the technique employed, nor of the training and reliability of the personnel who performed the task.

Research on the frequency range with which percussion seems to be the most effective began in the 1970s. Flower et al.[39] compared manual percussion with mechanical percussion and defined optimum frequencies as those which produced voice quivering. The recommended frequency in this study was 10 to

15 Hz. Clinically, 15 strokes per second equals 15 Hz. Mellins[71] states that a resonant frequency of 5 to 6 Hz is the optimum for mucus mobilization in adults. Sutton et al.[69] and Bateman et al.[72] used percussion with a frequency of 5 Hz.

Flower et al.[39] evaluated the performance of manual percussion by frequency. A range of 7.5 to 8.0 Hz was observed by physical therapists whose primary responsibilities were treating patients with pulmonary dysfunction. Therapists whose responsibilities included pulmonary patients but were not limited to this population used a percussion frequency of 6 Hz.

Hammon[73] compared manual percussion, mechanical percussion, and nontreatment in patients with alveolar proteinosis during bronchial lavage. They found that both types of percussion significantly improved the therapeutic results of bronchopulmonary lavage. Shunt fraction, however, improved more by manual percussion than by mechanical percussion or nontreatment. Maxwell and Redmond[74] studied the effects of manual percussion versus mechanical percussion operating at a frequency of 3.8 Hz. The efficacy was evaluated based on the volume of sputum produced by patients who were seated upright (45° angle) receiving treatment to the upper lobes. Before and after treatment, FEV_1 and forced vital capacity (FVC) values were also compared. There was no statistically significant difference between the mechanical and manual treatments. Denton[8] looked at the use of mechanical percussion with postural drainage versus postural drainage alone. Mechanical percussion was applied at a frequency of 20 to 45 Hz, which is above the optimal frequency recommended. Still, this high-frequency percussion was found to significantly increase the amount of sputum produced along with postural drainage.

What We Need to Know

The use of percussion within a treatment program increases the risks for developing intraventricular hemorrhage in infants,[56] yet adults seem to tolerate the techniques without difficulty.[48,49,57] Although the treatment includes more than just percussion, the question remains: are complications associated with the manual techniques (e.g., percussion) age related?

The more recent use of radioactive tracers to measure the velocity of the mucociliary transport system has allowed an objective measurement of centrally located mucous clearance that cannot be disputed. Its sole use as the endpoint in evaluating the efficacy of percussion is still questionable.

Sutton et al.[69] and Rossman et al.[70] reported that percussion did not increase the removal of radioactive tracers from central airways, yet it did increase the amount of sputum expectorated. In these two studies, the majority of the radioactive tracer was deposited in the more centrally located airways and, as Imle[50] states, perhaps the more patent airways. The addition of percussion to an existing treatment program was demonstrated to be no more effective in the removal of these tracers. Inherent in the performance of percussion is the objective of secretion clearance from a dysfunctional lung segment, not from the central airways or from those airways that are patent and functioning well. The increased amount of secretions expectorated by the subjects of both these studies may demonstrate the ability of percussion to remove sputum from the more peripheral airways that were not tagged by the aerosolized radioactive tracers. Bateman et al.[72] used a treatment of percussion, shaking, vibration, cough, and postural drainage, and found no increase in the clearance of tagged particles from the central airways when compared to the control group (postural drainage and cough). An increase in clearance of tagged particles from the *peripheral* airways was found. The percussion technique was not isolated, so the benefit to the peripheral airways cannot be attributed to percussion alone.

Regional lung studies on mucus transport velocities are needed in order to document the changes specific to the lung segments being treated.

Percussion requires continuous evaluation to optimize its performance. A discrepency exists among researchers with regard to the optimal treatment frequency for percussion. Different optimal frequencies may exist for different populations. Once the appropriate frequency is determined, physical therapists could provide percussion at that optimal frequency. Also, mechanical percussors could be evaluated for their efficacy during patient-performed therapy.

The optimal force of percussion is still difficult to assess. Flower et al.[39] measured forces of 58 to 65 kg/m/sec^2 (newtons). Other authors have reported the weight of the mechanical percussing devices, but a force readout was lacking. This seems to be another area requiring further investigation.

There is also no consistency among authors regarding the duration required to optimally perform percussion. The duration of reported percussive sessions varies in the literature from 20 to 30 seconds of percussion interrupted by deep breathing and coughing,[64] to 10 minutes of uninterrupted percussion,[7] to treatment sessions containing percussion which lasted up to 110 minutes.[30] What is the optimal duration for percussion? Perhaps there is a point at which the efficacy of percussion peaks and any more or less time spent performing it would be of minimal benefit, or even detrimental. Zidulka et al.[7] found that the use of percussion for 10 minutes was found to cause atelectasis in anesthetized dogs with no lung pathologies. The optimal duration may vary according to patient population. A chronically stable patient may require a shorter—or maybe even longer—treatment time than an acutely ill patient. Perhaps time itself should not be the endpoint of therapy, but rather the clinically assessed physical signs of cleared breath sounds, more efficient minute ventilation, or cessation of clearing secretions. There needs to be a common endpoint to ensure that current research can be compared.

There is a final factor to consider on the subject of percussion duration. In some of the above-mentioned studies, when percussion was added to an already prescribed program (e.g., one of postural drainage and directed coughing), percussion did not always provide a statistically significant increase in end results. Chopra et al.[12] found that percussion was better than postural drainage or nontreatment for increasing tracheal mucosal clearance velocity. When percussion was added to postural drainage, there was an increase in tracheal mucus velocity, although it did not prove to be statistically significant. Considering the small sample size of this final phase of his experiment (three dogs), statistical significance may have been difficult to obtain. Is it feasible that the addition of percussion to a postural drainage treatment hastened the secretion removal, thereby decreasing the amount of treatment time (and therefore therapist's time) necessary to obtain the same desired result? Van der Schans et al.[68] had similar results with 20 minutes of the combination of manual percussion, breathing exercises, cough, and rest periods (1 minute each, repeated 5 times) in one postural drainage position. Looking at the raw data of the first 10 minutes, Van der Schans et al. reported that the experimental group with manual percussion showed a greater clearance of radioactive tracer from the peripheral airways. The study also showed that by the end of 50 minutes of therapy, both treatment programs (one with manual percussion and one without) were equally effective.

Is it possible that percussion would enhance postural drainage and that the time needed for a single treatment session could be reduced? Van der Schans et al. used one postural drainage position (anterobasilar segment of the lower lobes) and performed percussion over the ventral aspect of the thorax of patients with stable chronic airway obstruction. Is it possible that if the percussion were directly over the lung segment for which the patient was positioned, and that lung segment has known pathology, the results might prove the efficacy of percussion?

Summary

Percussion is effective in the removal of excessive secretions from the tracheobronchial wall. Future study is required to determine the role of percussion in peripheral secretion clearance. Percussion needs continuous evaluation to optimize its performance with respect to patient populations, frequency, force of performance, and optimal treatment duration. The cumulative effect of percussion in conjunction with the other manual chest physical therapy techniques needs to be determined. Perhaps a longitudinal study of the long-term effects of removing percussion from pulmonary care would give further insight into the effectiveness of the technique.

Shaking/Vibration

What We Do

Immediately following a deep inhalation, whether spontaneously or mechanically generated, *shaking* is a bouncing rib cage maneuver applied to the thorax throughout exhalation. Shaking is usually preceeded by percussion in the appropriate postural drainage position. Because this technique is externally applied to the thorax, the same relative precautions as with percussion should be considered prior its use.

Vibration is the isometric cocontraction of the therapist's upper extremities, producing a vibration that is transmitted from the therapist's hands to the patient's thorax during the expiration. However, vibration can also be performed with a mechanical device. It may be performed after percussion in the postural drainage position; it has been used in conjunction with augmented inspiration via manual resuscitators. Because there is little or no pressure placed on the thorax with the use of vibration, there are no precautions to its use.

The techniques described above represent both ends of a spectrum of compression to the thorax. Shaking is vigorous and sits at the upper end of the spectrum, while vibration is mild and resides at the lower end. There are many points between these two ends which are clinically used. The determination of the amount of compressive force applied is left to the therapist's discretion.

What We Know

Shaking has been bronchoscopically observed to hasten the removal of secretions tagged with radioactive tracers from the tracheobronchial tree.[3,50] Vibration has been demonstrated by visual observation to enhance cephalic mucociliary transport.[3] The effects of shaking and vibration are discussed in the following section, based on patient population, methods of evaluation, and performance of the technique.

Patient Population

Shaking and/or vibration has been studied more often in neonates than in adults. Finer et al.[75] compared the use of vibration alone to no treatment in intubated neonates. The group receiving the treatment of vibration had a significantly lower incidence of postextubation atelectasis and need for reintubation than their untreated counterparts.

Effectiveness Evaluation Methods

Secretion Production. Hammon and Martin[76] found that manual shaking was more effective than mechanical shaking during bronchopulmonary lavage in patients with alveolar proteinosis, although the results were not significant. Pavia et al.[34] found that mechanical vibration in a Trendelenberg position increased the amount of mucous clearance, though the difference from the control group (also in the Trendelenberg position) was not significant. Sutton et al.[69] also looked at tracheobronchial clearance in adults with chronic obstructive pulmonary disease (COPD) with excessive secretion production. The addition of vibratory shaking to a regimen of postural drainage increased the dry weight of secretions removed. Bateman et al.[72] found an increase in sputum volume removed during treatment (percussion, vibration, and shaking, with cough in postural drainage) when compared to postural drainage and cough alone.

Oxygenation. Holloway et al.,[67] Walsh et al.,[77] and Fox et al.[78] found that the use of vibration decreased oxygenation levels in neonates. The decreases in oxygenation in these studies were explained in many ways. Holloway et al.[67] could reverse the decrease in oxygenation by the use of hyperinflation. Fox et al.[78] attributed the changes in oxygenation to suctioning, rather than the performance of vibration. Gregory noted that oxygenation decreased during crying, but not when the child was quiet.[79] Handling of infants alone can result in an increase in oxygen uptake ($\dot{V}O_2$),[80] causing hypoxemia.[81]

In contrast, Curran and Kachoyeanos[82] showed that vibrations produced by an electrical toothbrush resulted in an increased PaO_2, as well as clearer breath sounds, in their neonatal population. Finer and Boyd[21] also found an increase in oxygenation with their treatment program, which included vibration.

Tudelhope and Bagley[65] and Raval et al.[66] all found no significant changes in oxygenation with the use of vibration. Their patient population also was neonates.

In an acutely ill adult population, Holody and Goldberg[28] found mechanical vibration in the upright positions increased the PaO_2 after 30 to 60 minutes. There was no significant change in the partial arterial pressure of carbon dioxide ($PaCO_2$) or in the pH during the same time period. Records of neither sputum production nor mechanical vibrator frequency were described in the study.

Mucociliary Transport Velocity.   King et al.[83] and Rubin et al.[84] found an increase in tracheal mucus flow in animal models. Pavia et al.[34] and Sutton et al.[69] showed an increase in the mucociliary transport velocity in the central airways that did not reach statistical significance when compared to their control treatment. Sutton et al. stated that "radioaerosol deposition patterns were predominantly central." Bateman et al.,[72] whose tracers were more uniformly distributed through the lungs, found no change in the clearance of central tracers when compared to cough alone. However, the treatment program consisting of percussion, postural drainage, vibration, and shaking was significantly more effective than cough alone in clearing the tracers from the intermediate and peripheral airways.

Performance of the Technique

The work of King et al.[83] on anesthetized dogs demonstrated that by using a chest wall vibrating frequency of 13 Hz, a dramatic increase in the tracheal mucus flow could be produced. Rubin et al.[84] evaluated two mechanical means of providing chest wall vibrations to anesthetized dogs. A commercially available vibrating pad (at 40 Hz) had no effect on the tracheal mucus velocity, while an experimental device (at 13 Hz) increased tracheal mucus velocity by 204 percent.

Sutton et al.[69] and Bateman et al.[72] used a frequency of 2 Hz for shaking and 12 to 16 Hz for vibration on human subjects. They found no significant changes in clearance from the central airways when compared to other treatments, but Bateman et al.[72] did find a difference in peripheral airway clearance rate. Pavia et al.[34] used a mechanical vibrator at a frequency of 41 Hz. There was no significant change in mucociliary transport velocity between the vibration trials and control trials.

High-Frequency Oscillations

High-frequency oscillations (ventilation) have been applied at the airway opening in an attempt to enhance mucous clearance from the tracheobronchial tree. George et al.[85] showed that in a normal population, orally applied symmetrical oscillations of 8 to 12 Hz provided an increase in mucociliary clearance. This clearance was more effective than cough alone in clearing radioisotopes from the tracheobronchial tree. Freitag et al.,[86] using the animal model, showed that high-frequency oscillations of 14 Hz at the airway opening provided an increase in mucus clearance. An evaluation of postural drainage alone showed an equal ability to provide an increase in mucus clearance. However, the combination of postural drainage and high-frequency oscillation was found to have a threefold increase in the mucus clearance over high-frequency oscillation or postural drainage alone. Van Hengstrum et al.[87] showed no difference in tracheobronchial clearance with a combination of oral high-frequency oscillations and huffing compared to a control group with huffing alone. Van Hengstrum's group used the individual subject's respiratory resonant frequency to perform the oral high-frequency oscillations. The frequency range was 9.2 to 25 Hz. In contrast, other investigators have found no change or even a downstream movement of mucus with the use of orally applied high-frequency oscillations.[85,88] At this time the procedure is considered experimental and has not been incorporated into clinical practice.

What We Need to Know

Shaking and vibration seem to be the least studied of the chest physical therapy techniques. Therapists empirically use shaking and vibration to enhance the mucus transport following percussion. If this is the outcome, regional mucus transport velocities within the areas treated could be measured to provide the answers about its effectiveness. Bateman et al.[72] did show peripheral secretion clearance, though treatment included percussion as well as shaking and vibration in postural drainage positions. Clinically, shaking and vibration are used in combination with percussion and postural drainage. Does shaking/vibration enhance the effects of postural drainage and percussion, or is it effective on its own merit? Does the inclusion of shaking and/or vibration reduce the treatment time needed to achieve the same results?

Vibration seems to be used primarily in pediatric and neonatal populations. Shaking is used more often in adult populations. What is the reason for these preferences? Is there an optimal frequency for each population of patients? King et al.[83] and Rubin et al.,[84] using animal models, found that a frequency of 13 Hz was effective to mobilize secretions while a frequency of 40 Hz was found to be ineffective. Bateman's and Sutton's groups used a frequency of 12 to 16 Hz for vibration and 2 Hz for shaking in adults. This frequency did not enhance mucociliary transport rates in the central airways when compared to controls, but did produce an increase in the mucociliary transport velocity from the peripheral lung regions in adults. Van Hengstrum et al.[87] found the respiratory system's resonant frequency for each individual in their study; the range was 9.2 to 25 Hz. Should the frequency of shaking mimic the optimal resonant frequency of the lung?

What is the optimal force for shaking? Is it different depending on the patient population? The stiffness of the thorax of a patient with COPD may indicate a different amount of force than that of an infant with pneumonia.

The use of oral high-frequency oscillations needs further investigation to determine the proper frequency in humans with respect to their disease state, and the most effective form of application. The practicality of high-frequency oscillations has yet to be shown.

Summary

Shaking and vibration appear to increase peripheral secretion clearance. Optimal guidelines need to be established with respect to patient populations on the frequency, intensity, and duration of shaking and vibration. The cumulative effect of shaking and vibration, in conjunction with the other manual techniques of chest physical therapy, needs to be determined. The clinical feasibility of oral high-frequency oscillations requires further study.

AIRWAY CLEARANCE

The purpose of the previously described manual techniques is to effectively assist in the removal of excessive secretions from the peripheral tracheobronchial tree and move them upstream—more toward the glottis. Once the secretions arrive at the subsegmental bronchi, they often can be effectively cleared by a cough. However, independent coughing is neither always possible nor the most effective in all patient populations. Variations on the cough technique, namely huff, tracheal stiumulation, FET, and assisted cough, are each used clinically for specific patient populations. When none of these procedures effectively clears the airway, suctioning may be necessary. In the following sections, cough, variations on the cough technique as well as suctioning will be discussed with regard to what we do, what we know, and what we need to know.

What We Do

Cough

A cough is produced by a coordinated effort made up of three phases: inspiration, compression, and expulsion.[89] The patient is asked to inhale deeply, close the glottis, create an increased intrathoracic pressure by contracting the abdominal and the expiratory muscles (bearing down), release the glottis, and finally expel the air while continually contracting the forced expiratory muscles. Expiratory flow rates during a cough can be as high as 70 mph.

Huff

A huff is a forced expiratory effort that is in many ways similar to the cough. The difference lies in the deletion of the compression stage (i.e., there is no glottis closure). The patient is asked to inhale deeply and rapidly contract the abdominal and expiratory muscles for a forced expiration through an open airway, as if to say, "Ha, ha, ha." Without the compression phase of a cough, a huff has been seen bronchoscopically to stabilize collapsible airway walls in patients with chronic airflow obstruction.[52]

Forced Expiration Technique

The performance of FET is characterized by one or two forced expirations from mid to low lung volumes, again eliminating the compression phase of a cough when used with controlled breathing exercises. FET is thought to "milk" the more peripheral airways of their secretions, making overall lung clearance more effective. FET has been used in patients with COPD, asthma, and cystic fibrosis.[53,54,87,89–92]

Tracheal Stimulation

Coughing, huffing, and FET require attention to and an understanding of the task at hand. Tracheal stimulation is a technique that can be used to facilitate the cough reflex in patients who might otherwise not be able to clear their airway independently or upon command, such as adult patients who are neurologically impaired or very young children. To perform this technique, the therapist's thumb or index finger is placed just above the suprasternal notch of the manubrium.[44] A quick pressure is applied over the trachea in a posterocaudal (down and in) direction. A rapid and forceful cough will follow. This technique should be reserved for patients who are unable to generate a cough on their own. It is not intended for a patient who is able but unwilling to cough.

Assisted Coughing

A forceful contraction of the expiratory muscles is essential to provide the increased intrathoracic pressure that powers the expulsion phase of coughing. When abdominal muscle function is decreased, the effectiveness of the cough is impaired. A manually assisted cough is used to increase the strength of the expulsion phase in patients who have insufficient abdominal musculature. Assisted coughing is most often performed on patients with spinal cord injuries.[93,94] Thus, assisted coughing is sometimes referred to as quad coughing because of its use with patients who have had spinal cord injuries resulting in quadraplegia. The therapist's fist is placed just below the xiphoid process, between the costocondral margins. Then the usual cough sequence occurs: the patient inhales deeply, closes the glottis, and as the expulsion phase begins, the therapist pushes inward and upward with a fist, maximizing the movement of the diaphragm during the cough. Because of the lack of sensation in patients with spinal cord injuries, this assist can be quite vigorous without concern for causing pain to the patient. An assisted cough is akin to the Heimlich maneuver, except the patient and therapist coordinate this procedure with the expulsion phase of the cough sequence.

Suctioning

Suctioning is the least desirable way to clear an airway. It is an invasive and potentially harmful means of clearing secretions and should be used only when all of the above mechanisms would fail to produce the desired results. For some patients, there is no alternative to suctioning. For example, intubated patients routinely need suctioning, since the tube negates their own mucociliary clearance.[95] The following is a protocol for suctioning.

1. *Equipment.* Suctioning apparatus set between -100 mmHg for children and -160 mmHg for adults,[96] with an appropriately sized suction catheter (internal diameter of endotracheal tube/2 = external diameter of the suction catheter)[97] attached to the suction tubing. Both a sterile glove and a clean glove must be available.

2. *Prepare the patient.* Pre-oxygenation, with supplemental oxygen by means of a face mask, a manual resuscitator bag, or a fraction of inspired oxygen (FiO_2) of 1.0 by the ventilator, should be considered prior to suctioning in any patient with hypoxemia, cardiac irregularities, or acute or chronic pulmonary diseases. If there is any potential for suctioning to result in clinically significant hypoxemia, preoxygenation prior to suctioning is warranted. Explain the procedure beforehand to the patient.

3. *Prepare the therapist.* Wash hands. Gloves should be worn on both hands to protect the therapist, although only one glove needs to be sterile. Protective eye wear and mask should also be worn, since there is a danger of exposure of the therapist's mucus membranes to secretions from infected patients.

4. *Procedure.*
   a. Slide catheter out of packaging, using the sterile gloved hand. Since the catheter will come in contact with the trachea, sterility is important. The clean gloved hand will do all of the "dirty" work.
   b. Remove supplemental oxygen device, if used, with clean hand.
   c. Insert catheter into airway (nasally, orally, or tracheally) with the sterile hand. The catheter's suction port remains open while the catheter is passed into the airway.

    d. Once the catheter is inserted fully and the carina (a point of resistance) is felt, the catheter should be pulled back slightly to avoid any damage to the carina.

    e. Apply suction by occluding the suction port with the clean gloved thumb as the catheter is being rotated, and slowly remove it from the airway. Suction should be applied for 15 seconds or less during the removal of the catheter from the trachea.[98,99]

5. *Attention to the patient.* Re-administer supplemental oxygen to the patient if appropriate. If repeated suctioning is required, allow for a return to respiratory baseline prior to repeating the suction protocol.

6. *Attention to the therapist.* The soiled sterile glove should be pulled off inside-out and placed into the clean gloved hand. This clean glove is then removed by turning it inside-out (keeping the sterile glove within), and placed along with the mask in an appropriate waste receptical. Eyewear and hands should be washed before the therapist leaves the patient's room.

What We Know

Cough

Mucus clearance is accomplished in health by the normal mucociliary transport system. When the system is functioning properly, there is little need to cough.[100] In patients with altered or overwhelmed mucociliary transport systems, cough becomes both a powerful supplemental clearing and a protective mechanism.[100,101]

Mechanics. A cough is produced by a coordinated effort made up of three phases: inspiration, compression, and expulsion. The inspiratory phase begins with the contraction of the abductor muscles of the arytenoid cartilages. This contraction widens the opening between the vocal cords and permits the rapid inhalation of 1 to 2 L of air.

The compression phase of the cough begins with the action of the adductor muscles of the arytenoid cartilages, closing of the glottis. The contractions of the expiratory muscles during this phase force the diaphragm upward, creating a high intrathoracic pressure of up to 200 mmHg. These high pressures dynamically compress the tracheobronchial tree, thus decreasing the cross-sectional area of the airways and increase the linear velocity of airflow.

The expulsive phase of the cough begins with the opening of the glottis, promoting the rapid velocity of air out of the lungs. The forced contraction of the expiratory muscles continues throughout the expulsion phase to maintain high expiratory flow rates. The decreased cross-sectional area of the airways also helps to maintain the high velocity of the expired air.

Effectiveness. Leith states that cough effectiveness is dependent upon the intrathoracic volume.[100] Since body position influences lung volume (see Ch. 5), cough effectiveness has been evaluated according to position. Curry and Van Eeden[13] studied air flow during coughing in normal subjects in various positions.

Upright sitting, which produces the highest lung volume, was found to produce the highest expiratory flow rates. Starr[17] and Yamazaki et al.[102] studied positional effectiveness of cough in postoperative patients. The upright sitting position was again found to produce the greatest expiratory flow rates and the highest intrapleural pressures.

Cough effectiveness is also dependent upon the decreased cross-sectional area of the airways, which helps maintain the high velocity of the expired air. A pressure gradient is created between the upper airways, which are at atmospheric pressure, and the alveoli, which are at a high intrathoracic pressure. Proximal airway compression occurs up to the point where the flow of air out of the alveoli is balanced by the compression pressure acting upon the airway. This point of compression is called the flow limiting segment (FLS), or choke point, and occurs at different places within the airway at different lung volumes. At high lung volumes, the FLS probably lies within the trachea or mainstem bronchi. As lung volume decreases, the FLS moves distally, toward the alveoli. Although a movable point in the airway, the FLS is thought not to travel more distally than the sixth or seventh generation of the tracheobronchial tree. Smaldone and Smith[18] found that the FLS did not exceed the proximal subsegmental bronchi, even at lung volumes that approached residual volume (RV).

The FLS is dependent upon both the elastic properties of the lung and lung volume. Elastic recoil properties change with age and disease state; therefore, the effectiveness of a cough changes among different populations, from health to dysfunction, and in pediatric, adult, and geriatric patients.

Role in Treatment. The role of cough in the treatment of lung disease has been compared to a chest physical therapy routine of postural drainage, percussion, shaking, and coughing. Bain et al.[103] studied cough alone versus a combination of postural drainage, vibration, percussion, and coughing in patients with an acute exacerbation of cystic fibrosis. There was an improvement, measured by pulmonary function test (PFT) results and sputum characteristics, in both groups over a two-week period; however, one group was not significantly different from the other. DeBoeck[104] showed no significant short-term difference in pulmonary function studies or sputum production when cough alone was compared to the combination of postural drainage, percussion, and vibration with cough in nine patients with stable cystic fibrosis.

Oldenberg et al.[35] evaluated the role of coughing, postural drainage without coughing, and exercise on the removal of radioaerosolized droplets in patients with chronic bronchitis. The patients had a wide variation in volume of sputum expectorated, from 10 to 120 ml/day. Cough alone proved to be the most effective method of removing the tracer. In this study, particle distribution was greatest in the central airways, indicating that cough was most effective in clearing the central airways. Bateman et al.[72] studied cough alone versus cough and a combination of manual techniques in patients with chronic bronchitis and bronchiectasis. Once again, cough was as successful as the combination in the removal of the centrally located tracer. However, peripheral mucociliary clearance and overall sputum production increased in the group that received the manual techniques. Sutton et al.[54] studied 10 patients, all of whom had increased secretions (63 ml/day), to evaluate secretion removal manuevers and assess their efficacy. The methodology in this study consisted of a control group, a cough group, group performing FET, and a group performing FET during postural drainage. Coughing was not found to be as effective in clearing a radioaerosolized tracer as FET or FET with postural drainage.

Huff

The intrathoracic pressures that create the decrease in the cross-sectional area of the tracheobronchial tree and produce the FLS in health, act differently in the diseased airways of patients with COPD. The airways in COPD have decreased supporting structures, and rather than being compressed by the intrathoracic pressure, they actually become collapsed. By trapping the air behind the closed airway, the forced expulsion of air during a cough is ineffective in clearing secretions. The huff manuever, when compared to a cough, has been shown to produce a larger volume of exhaled gas at a higher flow rate in patients with chronic airflow obstruction.[52] This may mean that huffing is potentially more effective than coughing for secretion removal in patients with collapsible airways.

Techniques similar to the huff have also been described and evaluated. Sackner and Kim[1] reported that periodic airflow at an expiratory velocity that is greater than inspiratory velocity (similar to the huff) is effective in propelling secretions downstream. The long-term (3 years) effect of another forced expiratory maneuver similar to a huff was compared to a regimen of postural drainage, percussion, vibration, and coughing by Reisman et al.[41] The forced expiratory maneuver was described as (1) two maximal inspirations, each followed by a prolonged controlled forced expiration, and then (2) three normal quiet inspirations, each followed by a prolonged controlled forced expiration. A minimum of three coughs were then performed. Patients who performed this forced expiratory maneuver alone were found to have significantly greater annual rate of decline in mid-expiratory flow rate ($FEF_{25-75\%}$), FEV_1, and Shwachman clinical score. The authors' findings concluded in favor of continuing a routine chest physical therapy session rather than independent coughing alone. A word of clarification on this last study. The forced expiratory maneuver described by Reisman et al. is not the FET described by Pryor et al.,[53] Sutton et al.,[54] Clarke,[90] and Verboon et al.[105]

Forced Expiration Technique

Large lung volumes that usually precede a cough produce an FLS that lies fairly close to the glottis, perhaps within the trachea or the mainstem bronchi. This makes coughing very effective in clearing the central airways, but apparently of limited value in the peripheral airways. At lower lung volumes, the equal pressure point moves distally, incorporating more of the peripheral airways.

The FET, because of its performance from mid to low lung volumes, is thought to promote secretion removal from more than the central airways.

FET has been shown in some instances to be more effective than vigorous cough in the clearance of radioaerosol particles and in the sputum yield of severely obstructed patients with copious sputum production.[54] FET has also been shown to increase sputum expectoration when compared to routine chest physiotherapy in subjects with cystic fibrosis.[53] FET with postural drainage has been shown to be as effective as the combination of postural drainage, percussion, and directed coughing in terms of sputum production and mucociliary clearance of radioaerosolized particles.[92] The results of several studies suggest that a treatment program that can independently be performed (FET, breathing exercises, and postural drainage) is as effective in the short term as a routine chest physical therapy session.

Suctioning

The necessity of suctioning in certain instances is not in doubt. Of concern are the several significant complications associated with its use. Suctioning is well known for its ability to cause significant hypoxemia.[106–112] Other documented complications of suctioning are bradycardia,[113,114] tachycardia,[115] hypotension,[113] hypertension,[116] increased intracranial pressure,[116,117] atelectasis,[78,99,118–120] tracheal damage,[121–124] and nosocomial infections.[120,125]

Hypoxemia. Hypoxemia, a commonly occurring and frequently researched complication of suctioning, is caused by a number of concomitant situations. First, apnea—usually at low lung volumes—occurs during the suctioning technique. However, Rindfleisch and Tyler[98] and Boutros[108] showed that the decrease in oxygenation during suctioning exceeds the decrease due to apnea alone.

Second, suctioning results in the removal not only of secretions but also of air from the tracheobronchial tree. The fall in PaO_2 that occurs with suctioning is directly related to the duration of suctioning.[98,126] The duration of negative pressure should not exceed 15 seconds.[98,99]

A final aspect surrounding the development of hypoxemia is the level of PaO_2 prior to suctioning. Taylor and Waters[112] demonstrated that cardiac surgical patients who had a decrease in PaO_2 prior to suctioning, had a greater decrease during suctioning than those patients with a normal oxygenation. Kelly et al.[110] found that patients who had a presuctioning PaO_2 of less than 100 mmHg showed a statistically and clinically significant decrease in PaO_2 with suctioning. Those patients with a presuctioning PaO_2 of greater than 100 mmHg, although showing a statistically significant decrease in PaO_2 and SaO_2, did not show a clinically significant decrease in PaO_2 level.

Identifying those patients at risk for developing hypoxemia during suctioning could help minimize the untoward effects of this common procedure. Kelly et al.[110] found no correlation between the patient's presuctioning FiO_2 and their postsuction PaO_2. Chulay,[127] in her study using cardiac surgical patients, found that the presuctioning PaO_2: PAO_2 (partial alveolar oxygen pressure) was a reliable predictor of PaO_2 after suctioning.

By knowing the mechanisms that cause hypoxemia during suctioning, many researchers have looked toward ameliorating these dangers.[77,108,127–132] The type of ventilation as well as the choice of catheter used during suctioning may change the hypoxemic outcome of the procedure. Clinical practice presently uses a number of methods of ventilatory assistance during suctioning: hyperoxygenation, manual resuscitation to provide hyperinflation and hyperoxygenation, in-line suction port adapters, and oxygen insufflation catheters.

Hyperoxygenation (pre-oxygenation) has been evaluated for its ability to improve presuctioning PaO_2, thereby negating any clinically significant hypoxemia during suctioning. Walsh et al.[77] evaluated two groups of premature infants, one with no supplemental oxygen and another with enough oxygen added to bring $TcPO_2$ measurements to between 90 and 100 mmHg. Suctioning showed a clinically significant decrease in $TcPO_2$ to 40 mmHg or less without supplemental oxygen, but showed that $TcPO_2$ with supplemental oxygen remained above 40 mmHg. Kerem[107] showed similar results.

The use of a *manual resuscitator bag* has been employed to provide hyperoxygenation as well as hyperinflation prior to and following suctioning. Gold et al.[128] proved that 4 large breaths in 30 seconds was as beneficial as administering an FiO_2 of 1.0 for 5 minutes in spontaneously breathing postoperative patients who had no history of lung disease. Chulay,[127] in a study on mechanically ventilated postoperative cardiac surgical patients (positive end-expiratory pressure [PEEP] < 5 mmHg), found the administration of 5 hyperinflation ($1.5 \times$ tidal volume [Vt]) and hyperoxygenation (15 L/min O_2) breaths within 30 seconds before and after endotracheal suctioning increased the patient's postsuctioning PaO_2. These patients had no history of COPD. In a study by Preusser et al.,[129] both the mechanical resuscitator bag and a ventilator, using an FiO_2 of 1.0, effectively prevented postsuctioning hypoxemia in patients 3.5 hours after coronary artery bypass graft (CABG) surgery. These patients also had no history of COPD.

The use of hyperinflation and hyperoxygenation via a manual resuscitator bag was further assessed for its effect on abnormal lung function.[130] The manual resuscitator bag again prevented PaO_2 values from falling below control levels following endotracheal suctioning in sheep with normal lung function. However, in sheep with abnormal lung function, manual resuscitation did not maintain presuctioning PaO_2 values. Mechanical hyperinflation and hyperoxygenation provided by a second ventilator proved more effective, maintaining acceptable PaO_2 levels in the abnormal lung function group.

Hyperoxygenation, particularly high concentrations, has always been used with caution, especially in patients with the possibility of hypoxic drive. The use of lower concentrations of oxygen in this patient population was studied by Rogge et al.[131] Hyperinflation with an FiO_2 of 1.0 was compared to hyperinflation with oxygen support of 20 percent higher than the maintenance oxygen level in acutely ill COPD patients. Using a resuscitator bag, the investigators kept constant the frequency of hyperinflation (4 breaths/patient), the volume of the hyperinflation (1.5 × a Vt of 10 ml/kg), the duration of suctioning (10 seconds) and the frequency of suctioning (3 passes/session). They could show no difference in postsuctioning PaO_2 between the two O_2 concentrations.

The use of a manual resuscitator often necessitates removing the patient from the mechanical ventilator during the suctioning procedure. Disconnecting patients who require PEEP from mechanical ventilation causes an immediate fall in PaO_2[133,134] The use of *an in-line suction port adaptor* placed in the ventilatory tubing or a closed endotracheal suction system allows the suctioning procedure to be performed without disconnecting the patient from the ventilator. The ease of this type of protocol and the maintenence of Vt, PEEP, and FiO_2 during the suction procedure are attractive. This type of suctioning protocol has met with favor by a number of authors.[115,132,135–140]

There are potential dangers with in-line suction systems. Suctioning removes not only secretions but also air from the lungs. Difficulties arise when inspiratory flow rates from the ventilator are less than suctioning flow rates.[108] Negative airway pressure within the lungs can potentially prevent the maintenance of O_2 level or PEEP, or cause atelectasis and hypoxemia.[140] The control and assist modes of mechanical ventilation used with adults, because of their lack of continuous flow rates and reserve, are cited as contributing to the untoward effects of in-line suctioning systems.[140] The low flow rates used with neonatal ventilators may also pose difficulties with the in-line port adaptors.[103] Another complication can occur if the port is not completely occlusive. A loss of mechanically delivered volume and/or pressure can occur, making ventilation inadequate.

Some ventilators are equipped with suction options: (1) the manual assist option delivers a hyperinflation breath to the patient by the mere push of a button, and (2) the O_2 for suctioning option increases the FiO_2 to 1.0 for a controlled period of time (about 2 minutes) in order to provide hyperoxygenation. Stone states that hyperoxygenation and hyperinflation delivered via the ventilator is equal to or superior to hyperinflation and hyperoxygenation using the manual resuscitator bag method.[141] There is a time delay between when the change to 100 percent is made and when the FiO_2 is actually delivered to the patient, based on the wash-out time of the ventilator tubing and the microprocessing of the ventilator itself.[142,143] Changing the ventilatory settings of a mechanical ventilator to achieve hyperoxygenation and hyperventilation is a dangerous proposition. It is a very real possibility that the patient will not be returned to the baseline ventilatory settings, in which case hyperinflation, and hyperoxygenation could continue long after the suctioning technique is over.

Oxygen insufflation catheterization during the suctioning procedure has been used in hopes of diminishing postsuctioning hypoxemia. A double lumen catheter is inserted into the trachea. One port delivers oxygen, while the other port is attached to suction. Kelly et al.[110] compared conventional single lumen suctioning to oxygen insufflation suctioning. All patients were anesthetized and paralyzed prior to undergoing cardiac surgery. Conventional suctioning showed a significant fall from baseline. Oxygen insufflation through the suction catheter produced a significant increase of 5 mmHg in PaO_2. There were no hyperinflation or hyperoxygenation procedures performed prior to or following suctioning.

Bradychardia and Tachycardia.   Although hypoxemia is the most commonly researched hazard of suctioning, other complications of the suctioning technique have been demonstrated. Cardiovascular changes have been reported due to parasympathetic stimulation and hypoxemia. Winston et al.[113] evaluated six adults who were intubated and mechanically ventilated patients. These patients had a reproducible 20 percent or greater fall in resting heart rate (HR) during endotracheal suctioning. Hypotension was noted in half of the subjects. Patients with an acute spinal cord injury also seem to respond with the vasovagal reflex of bradycardia and hypotension during suctioning.[114] Clarke et al., however, showed that there was an increase in heart rate with suctioning.[115]

Increased Intracranial Pressure.   Durand et al.,[116] using a suction adaptor, studied preterm infants, showing that endotracheal suctioning increases blood pressure, intracranial pressure, and cerebral perfusion pressure, all implicators in the pathogenesis of intracranial hemorrhage. These changes may be produced by an increase in intrathoracic pressure, thus impeding venous return and increasing cerebral venous pressure. Similar results were reported by Fanconi and Duc.[117]

Walsh et al. showed a decrease in the mixed venous oxygen saturation ($S\bar{v}O_2$) with endotracheal suctioning.[109] This change was felt to be due to an increase in oxygen uptake ($\dot{V}O_2$), with an inadequate rise or, in some cases, a fall in cardiac output ($\dot{Q}$) during suctioning. SaO_2 was found to be an insensitive indicator of changes occurring in $S\bar{v}O_2$.

Atelectasis.   The association between suctioning and resultant atelectasis is not well documented. Suctioning that produces subatmospheric pressure within the thorax can potentially cause atelectasis.[99,118] Hyperinflation after suctioning has been utilized in hopes of alleviating this possibility.[119] Fox et al.[78] found little evidence to support the presence of postsuctioning atelectasis, as there was no change in total lung–thorax compliance or functional residual capacity (FRC).

Tracheal Damage.   Tracheal damage is another complication of suctioning. Kleiber et al.[121] found that suctioning to a predetermined distance within the trachea, rather than inserting the suction catheter until resistance is felt, resulted in significantly less tracheal damage. Brodsky et al.[122] studied the microscopic pathology of the distal trachea in intubated low birth weight infants to determine if there was any correlation between tracheal pathology and tracheal suctioning. At autopsy, tracheal damage was present when uncontrolled deep suctioning was performed. The amount of tracheal pathology was diminished when suctioning was limited to the end of the artificial airway.

Kleiber et al. felt that the direct mechanical insult of the catheter to the airway seemed to be the cause of tracheal trauma as the application of suction had no effect on the amount of tracheal damage.[121] Kuzenski,[123] however, demonstrated that when a negative pressure of 200 mmHg was used, tracheal trauma was produced. A lesser amount of suction, 100 mmHg, was found to be effective, yet did not cause tracheal trauma. Jung and Gottleib[124] summarize by stating that repetition, vigor, and the amount of suction applied to the airway are all likely causes of tracheal trauma.

Nosocomial Infections. Nosocomial infections can occur if the sterile field is broken by the therapist or if the catheter is contaminated upon entering the nasal or oral cavity.[120] Sterile-sleeved catheters remove the need for sterile technique, thereby reducing the chance of nosocomial pneumonias.[125] However, the cost of these sleeved systems is reportedly 25 times higher than of sterile catheter and gloves. On a cost basis alone, it may be hard to justify their use.[136]

Suctioning Efficacy. The efficacy of suctioning has been researched to provide clinicians with some guidance in their protocol. Brown et al.[132] found that the flow rates recorded through the catheter during continuous suctioning were recorded at 18 to 29 L/min, but only 8 to 0 L/min when the interrupted technique was employed. It is thought that rotating the catheter during withdrawl from the trachea avails a larger surface area to the negative pressure, making suctioning more effective.

Saline is often instilled into a tracheal tube prior to the procedure suction. Three possible reasons have been given for its use: (1) to decrease the viscosity of the secretions, (2) to increase the cough, and (3) to lubricate the catheter.

Hanley et al.[144] determined that the majority of a 5 mm radioisotope–labeled bolus of saline injected through a tracheal tube remained within the trachea and the mainstem bronchi up to 30 minutes after the injection. Therefore, it is difficult to decrease mucus viscosity if the saline cannot reach the secretions. (Suctioning was only able to recover a maximum of 19 percent of the tagged saline, leaving the rest within the respiratory system.) Demers and Saklad[99] contend that mucous and saline will not mix even after vigorous shaking, again attacking the ideal of decreased viscosity. Ackerman[145] has denounced the use of saline for the purpose of thinning, mobilizing, or removing secretions.

Demers and Saklad[99] proposed that the main advantage of saline instillation was stimulation of a vigorous cough. The use of the suction catheter itself is enough stimulation to cough. The use of saline to meet the same end is at best a duplication of effort.

Since the instillation of saline is usually through an artificial airway—and the suction catheter is placed through the same airway—there is little need for a lubricant. When nasotracheal suctioning is performed, a water-soluble lubricant is used, making saline as a lubricant unnecessary.

What We Need to Know

Cough, Forced Expiration Technique, Huff, and Assisted Cough

Cough. Bateman et al.,[72] looking at immediate outcomes, showed that cough alone was equally effective in clearing radioactive particles from the central airways of patients with chronic bronchitis and bronchiectasis when compared to a treatment program including other manual chest physical therapy techniques. There is no disagreement that coughing is effective in removing centrally located droplets. Bateman et al. also found that the group receiving manual techniques along with cough cleared more secretions than the group performing cough alone. Oldenberg et al.[35] found cough to be an effective maneuver in clearing the peripheral lung regions in patients with chronic bronchitis. Not all of the subjects in that study had excessive secretions (range: 10 to 120 ml/day). The radioaerosolized particle distribution was predominantly located in the central airways, and the definition of peripheral zones was different from those described by Bateman et al.[72] Studies whose methodology maps the central airways will have the greatest information on the central airways, but perhaps not on the peripheral airways. Bateman et al., whose patients had a more uniform distribution of radioaerosolized tracer particles throughout the lungs, found a greater clearance in the peripheral and intermediate airways with his treatment program than with cough alone. The information regarding the role of cough in the peripheral airways seems conflicting.

DeBoeck,[104] studying the short-term outcomes, found the sole use of cough in patients with stable cystic fibrosis to be as effective as the combination of percussion, vibration, and cough in postural drainage positions. Efficacy was defined by measurements of FEV_1, peak expiratory flow rate, and lung volumes. The flow rates at high lung volumes, used to measure efficacy, may better reflect clearance from the larger airways, where cough alone is known to be effective. However, when more peripheral airways were studied the chest physiotherapy group had significantly higher test values for clearance. Again, the role of cough in the central airways is well known, but its role in the peripheral airways needs further study.

Another consideration in DeBoeck's study is the goal of therapy in the population used (patients with stable cystic fibrosis). The preventative nature of therapy means not necessarily short-term improvements but long-term stabilization of the disease progression. Reisman et al.[41] studied patients with stable cystic fibrosis to determine the long-term effects of the sole use of forced expiratory maneuver versus the combination of percussion, shaking, and cough in postural drainage positions. In view of the fact that the expiratory technique in the Reisman group's work was different than that in DeBoeck's research, it remains interesting that Reisman's long-term outcomes were not favorable, while DeBoeck found favorable short-term outcomes. Further studies could include the short-term effects of Reisman's forced expiratory maneuver, with special emphasis on the peripheral airways, and the long-term effects of DeBoeck's treatment program.

There have been patient populations that do not seem to benefit from secretion removal techniques during pulmonary dysfunction.[20] Some of these patients may benefit from a regimen of cough alone during a pulmonary dysfunction,[99] and others may patients benefit from a regimen consisting of the manual chest physical therapy techniques plus cough.[72] Further research is needed to determine the most effective and efficient treatment program for each patient population, based on patient age and disease process, as well as on available resources, time, and finances.

Forced Expiration Technique. Van Hengstum et al.[92] showed that the combination of FET, postural drainage, and breathing exercises was as effective as the combination of postural drainage, percussion, and directed coughing. Regional lung clearance was mapped by radioaerosolized particles. Central, intermediate, and peripheral lung fields were cleared equally by both treatment programs. Both Pryor et al.[53] and Sutton et al.[54] agree with these findings. The long-term outcomes of this treatment in place of conventional therapy also need to be researched.

Huff. Controversy exists as to the efficacy of the huff. FET has replaced the huff in many instances. However, the huff is still used for patients with tracheostomy tubes. The efficacy of the huff in this patient population is still in question. Could the FET be more effective with patients having tracheostomy tubes?

Assisted Cough. The assisted cough has not been adequately evaluated, although clinical use persists. Assisted cough needs to be researched to determine the optimal force to be provided by the therapist, the optimal position of the patient, and the procedure's efficacy when compared to other secretion removal techniques such as suctioning.

Suctioning

The complication of hypoxemia during suctioning is well documented. The best method for alleviating hypoxemia in different patient populations is not yet known. Spontaneously breathing patients have different needs than those patients being managed on mechanical ventilation, just as patients who are mechanically ventilated with PEEP have different needs than those who do not need PEEP, and those with underlying lung disease have different needs from those without lung disease.

Manual Resuscitator Bags. Manual resuscitator bags have been used to provide hyperinflation and hyperoxygenation in all of these populations, with differing results. The best method for hyperoxygenation and hyperinflation for each patient population needs to be examined, as does the cost effectiveness of each method.

Port Adapters and In-line Suctioning. Port adapters and in-line suctioning have allowed the patient to be suctioned and effectively supported without disconnection from the ventilator or alteration of settings. The in-line suctioning system could also negate the potential dangers of nosocomial infections. The cost of this type of system makes it prohibitive for most patients, however. The very ill patient who is suctioned every few hours, or the patient who is at high risk for nosocomial infections, may make the cost issue negligable. The same needs for maintenance of PEEP, FiO_2 Vt, and a sterile field exist in the pediatric populations, but low flow rates have made in-line suctioning hazardous. The question of the best means of suctioning the very ill infant remains unanswered.

Oxygen Insufflation. Oxygen insufflation seems to be one way of maintaining oxygenation during the suctioning procedures, but efficacy has not yet been determined. The size of the lumen of the suction port in the oxygen insufflation catheter is of concern. Since separate O_2 and suction tracts are housed within the same catheter, the lumen size of the suctioning port in the work of Bodai et al.[146] is smaller (12 French) than could otherwise be used (16 French). The effectiveness of suctioning was not addressed in the work done by Kelly et al.[110] The potential risks of repeated suctioning (trauma, bradycardia, tachycardia, hypotension, hypertension, and increased intracranial pressure) make oxygen insufflation of questionable benefit.

Spontaneously breathing patients can benefit from oxygen insufflation, but the mechanically ventilated, apneic patients may not. Spoerel and Chan[147] used a gas jet to deliver O_2 in the insufflation catheter, thereby providing O_2 to their patients who had suffered a head trauma but had no history of pulmonary disease. Suctioning was performed for 60 seconds. The PaO_2 values during a trial of suctioning without high-frequency jet oxygenation dropped to a low of 45 mmHg. With the use of high-frequency jet ventilation, a maintenance of arterial O_2 was demonstrated. Guntupalli et al.[148] also showed a maintenance of PaO_2 during the suctioning procedure with high-frequency jet ventilation. In the latter study, the high-frequency jet ventilation was housed within the endotracheal tube; therefore, there was no need to decrease the size of the suction catheter lumen.

Other Strategies for Handling Complications.   Studies focusing on other documented complications of suctioning have used somewhat extreme measures in order to correct them. Bradycardia and hypotension have been reversed with the parenteral delivery or nebulization of atropine.[113,114] Hypertension and increases in intracranial pressure in infants were reversed with muscle paralysis.[118] Increases in $\dot{V}O_2$ and inadequate compensation of $\dot{Q}$ continue to plague suctioning. Research focusing on less severe methods for ameliorating these complications must be pursued.

Suction Protocol.   The efficacy of suction protocol has not been determined. Is there a best method to employ when suctioning an airway? Intermittent suctioning versus rotation of the catheter has been studied for the effects on negative flow rates and tracheal trauma development. Could intermittent suctioning that begins with a higher flow rate but results in flow rates at the catheter tip equal to those found by rotating the catheter provide an effective means of suctioning without the tracheal damage?

Suctioning Duration.   What is the most effective suctioning time? Rindfleisch and Tyler observed that clinicians spend anywhere from 3 to 13 seconds occluding the suction port.[99] Spoerel and Chan suctioned their patient for 60 seconds.[147] Is it more effective to suction for short periods of time with repeated passes of the catheter or is it more advantageous to remain in the airway a bit longer to reduce the number of suctioning bouts?

Suctioning Efficacy.   How is efficacy determined? The amount of secretions removed? the dry weight of secretions removed? the improvement of breath sounds or arterial blood gas values? chest radiographic improvement? Bostick and Wendelgass evaluated the efficacy of saline instillation by postsuctioning PaO_2 levels. There was no statistical difference in arterial oxygenation found with or without the saline.[149] If improved oxygenation is one of the goals of suctioning, then saline instillation did not benefit the procedure. The weight of secretions was higher in the saline instillation group, but the amount of saline within the secretions was not accounted for. If the amount of secretions is one of the goals of suctioning, then an accurate account of the secretions removed is necessary. Perhaps, if improved alveolar $\dot{V}e$ is the goal of suctioning, then $PaCO_2$ would be a better indicator of suctioning efficacy.

SUMMARY

The evaluation of chest physical therapy manual techniques and of the methods of airway clearance have been researched, providing a great deal of useful information. However, questions regarding their efficacy, performance, and consequences remain. A more unified approach to the research of secretion removal would make a comparison of methods more clinically useful.

REFERENCES

1. Sackner M, Kim C: Phasic flow mechanisms of mucus clearance. Eur J Respir Dis, suppl. 71: S159, 1987
2. Wong J, Keen S, Wannamaker E et al: The effects of gravity on tracheal mucus transport rates in normal subjects and in patients with cystic fibrosis. Pediatrics 60:146, 1977
3. Kigin C: Advances in Chest Physical Therapy. American College of Chest Physicians, Park Ridge, IL, 1984
4. Anthonisen P, Riis P, Søgaard-Anderson T: Value of lung physiotherapy in treatment of acute exacerbations in chronic bronchitis. Acta Med Scand 175:715, 1964
5. Reines H, Sade R, Bradford B, et al: Chest physiotherapy fails to prevent postoperative atelectasis in children after cardiac surgery. Ann Sur 195:451, 1982
6. Huber A, Eggleston P, Morgan J: Effect of chest physiotherapy in asthmatic children, abstracted. J Allergy Clin Immunol 53:109, 1974
7. Zidulka A, Chrome J, Wight D et al: Clapping or percussion causes atelectasis in dogs and influences gas exchange. J Appl Physiol 66:2,833, 1989
8. Denton R: Bronchial secretions in cystic fibrosis: the effects of treatment with mechanical percussion vibration. Am Rev Respir Dis 86:41, 1962
9. Gaskel D, Webber B: The Brompton Hospital Guide to Chest Physiotherapy. Blackwell Scientific Publications, Oxford, 1973
10. Lorin M, Denning C: Evaluation of postural drainage by measurement of sputum volume and consistency. Am J Phys Med 50:215, 1971
11. Tecklin J, Holsclaw D: Evaluation of bronchial drainage in patients with cystic fibrosis. Phys Ther 55:1,081, 1975
12. Chopra S, Taplin G, Simmons D: Effects of Hydration and Physical Therapy on Tracheal Transport Velocity. Am Rev Respir Dis 115:1,009, 1977
13. Curry L, Van Eeden C: The influence of posture on the effectiveness of coughing. S Afr J Physiol 33:8, 1977
14. Kang B, Rogers L, Niederhuber S et al: Evaluation of postural drainage with percussion in chronic obstructive pulmonary disease, abstracted. J Allergy Clin Imm 53:109, 1974

15. Mazzacco M, Owens G, Kirilloff L et al: Chest percussion and postural drainage in patients with bronchiectasis. Chest 88:360, 1985

16. Ward R, Sanziger P, Bonica J et al: An evaluation of postoperative respiratory maneuvers. Surg Gynecol Obstet 123:51, 1966

17. Starr J: The influence of posture and cummulative trials on the effectiveness of coughing in the postoperative cholecystectomy patients. Unpublished thesis, Boston University, 1980

18. Smaldone G, Smith P: Location of flow limiting segments via airway catheters near residual volume in humans. J Appl Physiol 59:502, 1985

19. Wollmer P, Ursing K, Midgren B et al: Ineffeciency of chest percussion in the physical therapy of chronic bronchitis. Eur J Respir Dis 66:233, 1985

20. Graham W, Bradley D: Efficacy of chest physiotherapy and intermittent positive pressure breathing in the resolution of pneumonia. N Engl J Med 299:624, 1978

21. Finer N, Boyd J: Chest physiotherapy in the neonate: a controlled study. Pediatrics 61:282, 1978

22. Crane L, Zombek M, Krauss A, et al: Comparison of chest physiotherapy techniques in infants with HMD, abstracted. Pediatr Res 12:559, 1978

23. March H: Appraisal of postural drainage for chronic obstructive pulmonary disease. Arch Phys Med Rehab 11:528, 1971

24. May D, Munt P: Physiologic effects of chest percussion and postural drainage in patients with stable chronic bronchitis. Chest 75:29, 1979

25. Cochrane G, Webber B, Clarke S: Effects of sputum on pulmonary function. Br Med J 2:1,181, 1977

26. Feldman J, Traver G, Taussig L: Maximal expiratory flow after postural drainage. Am Rev Respir Dis 119:239, 1979

27. Campbell A, O'Connell J, Wilson F: The effect of chest physiotherapy upon the FEV_1 in chronic bronchitis. Med J Aust 1:33, 1975

28. Holody B, Goldberg H: The effects of mechanical vibration physiotherapy on arterial oxygenation in acutely ill patients with atelectasis or pneumonia. Am Rev Respir Dis 124:372, 1981

29. Connors A, Hammon W, Martin R et al: Chest physical therapy: the immediate effect on oxygenation in acutely ill patients. Chest 78:559, 1980

30. Mackenzie C, Shin B, McAslan T: Chest physiotherapy: the effect on arterial oxygenation. Anesth Analg 57:28, 1978

31. McDonell T, McNicholas W, FitzGerald M: Hypoxaemia during chest physiotherapy in patients with cystic fibrosis. Ir J Med Sci 345, 1986

32. Lord G, Herbert C, Francis D: A clinical, radiologic and physiologic evaluation of chest physiotherapy. J Maine Med Assoc 63:142, 1972

33. Bateman J, Duant K, Newman S et al: Regional lung clearance of excessive bronchial secretions during chest physiotherapy in patients with stable chronic airflow obstruction. Lancet 1:294, 1979

34. Pavia D, Thomson M, Phillipakos D: A preliminary study of the effect of a vibrating pad on bronchial clearance. Am Rev Respir Dis 113:92, 1976

35. Oldenberg F, Dolovich M, Montgomery J et al: Effects of postural drainage, exercise and cough on mucus clearance in chronic bronchitis. Am Rev Respir Dis 120:739, 1979

36. Mackenzie C, Shin B, Hadi F et al: Changes in total lung/thorax compliance following chest physiotherapy. Anesth Analg 59:207, 1980

37. Thoren L: Postoperative pulmonary complications: observations on their prevention by means of physiotherapy. Acta Chir Scand 107:193, 1954

38. Cerny F: Relative effects of bronchial drainage and exercise for inhospital care of patients with cystic fibrosis. Phys Ther 69:633, 1989

39. Flower K, Eden R, Lomax L: A new mechanical aid to physiotherapy in cystic fibrosis. Br Med J 2:630, 1979

40. Weller P, Bush E, Preece M et al: Short term effects of chest physiotherapy on pulmonary function in children with cystic fibrosis. Respiration 40:53, 1980

41. Reisman J, Rivington-Law B, Corey M et al: Role of conventional physiotherapy in cystic fibrosis. J Pediatr 113:632, 1988

42. Shapiro B, Harrison R, Trout C: Clinical Application of Respiratory Care. 2nd Ed. Yearbook Medical Publishers, Chicago, 1979

43. Zadai C: Physical therapy in the acutely ill medical patient. Phys Ther 61:1,746, 1981

44. Frownfelter D: Chest Physical Therapy and Pulmonary Rehabilitation. 2nd Ed. Yearbook Medical Publishers, Chicago, 1986

45. Starr J: Management of the Pulmonary Patient. American Physical Therapy Association, Arlington, VA, 1991

46. Humberstone N: Respiratory assessment and treatment. p. 283. In Irwin S, Tecklin J (eds): Cardiopulmonary Physical Therapy. 2nd Ed. CV Mosby, Philadelphia, 1990

47. Ciesla N, Rodrigues A, Anderson P et al: Incidence of extrapleural hematoma in patients with rib fractures receiving chest physical therapy, abstracted. Phys Ther 67:766, 1987

48. Hammon W, Kirmeyer P, Connors A et al: Effects of bronchial drainage on intracranial pressure in acute neurologic injuries, abstracted. Phys Ther 51:735, 1981

49. Brimioulle S, Moraine J, Kahn R: Passive physical therapy and respiratory therapy effects on intracranial pressure, abstracted. Crit Care Med 16:449, 1988

50. Imle P: Percussion and vibration. p. 81. In Mackenzie C, Imle P, Ciesla N (eds): Chest Physiotherapy in the Intensive Care Unit. 2nd Ed. Williams & Wilkins, Baltimore, 1989

51. Langlands J: The dynamics of cough in health and in chronic bronchitis. Thorax 22:88, 1967

52. Hietpas B, Roth R, Jensen W: Huff coughing and airway patency. Respir Care 24:710, 1979

53. Pryor J, Webber B, Hodson M: Evaluation of the forced expiration technique as an adjunct to postural drainage in treatment of cystic fibrosis. Br Med J 2:417, 1979

54. Sutton P, Parker R, Webber B et al: Assessment of the forced expiration technique, postural drainage and directed coughing in chest physiotherapy. Eur J Respir Dis 64:62, 1983

55. Hammon W, Martin R: Fatal pulmonary hemorrhage associated with chest physical therapy. Phys Ther 59:1,247, 1979

56. Raval D, Yeh T, Mora H et al: Chest physiotherapy in preterm infants with respiratory distress syndrome in the first 24 hours of life. J Perinatol 7:301, 1987

57. McQuillian K: The effects of Trendelenberg position for postural drainage on cerebrovascular status in head injured patients, abstracted. Heart Lung, 16:327, 1987

58. Wood D, Kraves L, Lecks H: Physical therapy for children with intractable asthma. J Asthma Res 7:177, 1970

59. Webber B: Current trends in the treatment of asthma. Physiotherapy 59:388, 1973

60. Etches M, Scott B: Chest physiotherapy in the newborn: effect on secretions removed. Pediatrics 62:713, 1978

61. Newton D, Stevenson A: Effect of physiotherapy on pulmonary function. Lancet: 2:228, 1978
62. Mackenzie C: Physiological changes following chest physiotherapy. p. 216. In Mackenzie C, Imle P, Ciesla N: Chest Physiotherapy in the Intensive Care Unit. 2nd Ed. Williams & Wilkins, Baltimore, 1989
63. Murray J: The ketchup bottle method, editorial. N Engl J Med 300:1,155, 1979
64. Murphy M: Chest percussion: help or hinderance to postural drainage. Ir Med J 76:189, 1983
65. Tudelhope D, Bagley C: Techniques of physiotherapy in intubated babies with the respiratory distress syndrome. Aust Paediatr J 16:226, 1980
66. Raval D, Yeh T, Mora H et al: Changes in transcutaneous PO_2 during tracheobronchial hygiene in neonates. Perinatology/Neonatology 4:41, 1980
67. Holloway R, Adams E, Desai S et al: Effect of chest physiotherapy on blood gases of neonates treated by intermittent positive pressure respiration. Thorax 24:421, 1969
68. Van der Schans C, Piers D, Postma D: Effect of manual percussion on tracheobronchial clearance in patients with chronic airflow obstruction and excessive tracheobronchial secretion. Thorax 41:448, 1986
69. Sutton P, Lopez-Vidriero M, Pavia D et al: Assessment of percussion, vibratory shaking, and breathing exercises in chest physiotherapy. Eur J Respir Dis 66:147, 1985
70. Rossman C, Waldes R, Sampson D, et al: Effects of chest physiotherapy on the removal of mucous in patients with cystic fibrosis. Am Rev Respir Dis 126:131, 1982
71. Mellins R: Pulmonary physiotherapy in the pediatric age group. Am Rev Respir Dis 110:137, 1974
72. Bateman J, Newman SD, Daunt K et al: Is cough as effective as chest physiotherapy in the removal of excessive tracheobronchial secretions? Thorax 36:682, 1981
73. Hammon W: Manual versus mechanical percussion for clearance of alveolar contents, abstracted. Phys Ther 63:756, 1983
74. Maxwell M, Redmond A: Comparative trial of manual and mechanical percussion technique with gravity assisted bronchial drainage in patients with cystic fibrosis. Arch Dis Child 54:542, 1979
75. Finer N, Moriartey R, Boyd J et al: Post extubation atelectasis: a retrospective review and a prospective controlled study. J Pediatr 94:110, 1979
76. Hammon W, Martin R: Percussion versus vibration for clearance of alveolar contents, abstracted. Phys Ther 60:589, 1980
77. Walsh C, Bada H, Korones S et al: Controlled supplemental oxygenation during tracheobronchial hygiene. Nurs Res 36:211, 1987
78. Fox W, Schwartz J, Shaffer T: Pulmonary physiotherapy in neonates: physiologic changes and respiratory management. J Pediatr 92:977, 1978
79. Gregory G: Respiratory care of the child. Crit Care Med 8:582, 1980
80. Yeh T, Leu S, Pyati S et al: Changes in O_2 consumption ($\dot{V}O_2$) in response to NICU care procedures in premature infants, abstracted. Pediatr Res 16:315, 1982
81. Long J, Philip A, Laucey J: Excessive handling as a cause of hypoxemia. Pediatrics 65:203, 1980
82. Curran C, Kachoyeanos M: The effects on neonates of two methods of chest physical therapy. MCN 4:309, 1979
83. King M, Phillips D, Gross D et al: Enhanced tracheal mucus clearance with high frequency chest wall compression. Am Rev Respir Dis 128:511, 1983

84. Rubin E, Scantlin G, Chapman G et al: The effects of chest wall oscillations on mucus clearance: comparison of two vibrators. Pediatr Pulmonol 6:122, 1989

85. George R, Johnson M, Pavia D et al: Increase in mucociliary clearance in normal man induced by oral high frequency oscillation. Thorax 40:433, 1985

86. Freitag L, Long W, Kim C et al: Removal of excessive bronchial secretions by asymmetric high frequency oscillations. J Appl Physiol 67:614, 1989

87. Van Hengstrum M, Festen J, Beurskens C et al: No effect of oral high frequency oscillation combined with forced expiration manouevers on tracheobronchial clearance in chronic bronchitics. Eur Resp J 3:14, 1990

88. McEvoy R, Davies N, Hedenoterna G: Lung mucociliary transport during high frequency ventilation. Am Rev Respir Dis 126:452, 1982

89. Irwin R, Rosen M, Braman S: Cough: a comprehensive review. Arch Intern Med 137:1,186, 1977

90. Clarke S: Management of mucus hypersecretion. Eur J Respir Dis, suppl. 71:S136, 1987

91. Pavia D: The role of chest physiotherapy in mucus hypersecretion. Lung suppl. 168:S614, 1990

92. Van Hengstrum M, Festen J, Beurskens C et al: Conventional physiotherapy and forced expiration technique manoeuvres have similar effects on tracheobronchial clearance. Eur Respir J 1:758, 1988

93. Kocan M: Pulmonary considerations in the critical care phase. Crit Care Nurs Clin North Am 2: 369, 1990

94. Siebeens A, Kirby N, Puolos D: Cough following transections of spiral cord at C6. Arch Phys Med Rehabil 45:1, 1964

95. Tenaillon A, Boiteau R, Perrin-Gachadoat D et al: Humidification and aspiration of the respiratory tract in patients with mechanical ventilation, abstracted. Rev Prat 40:2,315, 1990

96. Imle P, Klemic N: Methods of airway clearance: coughing and suctioning. In Mackenzie C, Imle R, Ciesla N (eds): Chest Physiotherapy in the Intensive Care Unit. 2nd Ed. Williams & Wilkins, Baltimore, 1989

97. Rosen M, Hillard E: The effects of suction in clinical medicine. Br J Anaesth 32:486, 1960

98. Rindfleish S, Tyler M: Duration of suctioning: an important variable. Respir Care 28: 457, 1983

99. Demers R, Saklad M: Mechanical aspiration: a reappraisal of its hazards. Respir Care 20:661, 1975

100. Leith D: Cough. Phys Ther 48:439, 1968

101. Camner P, Mossberg B, Phillipson G et al: Elimination of test particles from the human tracheobronchial tree by voluntary coughing. Scand J Respir Dis 60:56, 1979

102. Yamazaki S, Owaga J, Shohzu A et al: Intrapleural cough pressure in patients after thorocotomy. J Thorac Cardiovasc Surg 80:600, 1980

103. Bain J, Bishop J, Olinsky A: Evaluation of directed coughing in cystic fibrosis. Br J Dis Chest 82:138, 1988

104. DeBoeck C: Cough versus chest physiotherapy-a comparison of the acute effects on pulmonary function in patients with cystic fibrosis. Am Rev Respir Dis 129:182, 1984

105. Verboon J, Bakker W, Sterk P: The value of the forced expiration technique with and without postural drainage in adults with cystic fibrosis. Eur J Respir Dis 69:169, 1986

106. Peterson G, Pierson D, Hunter P: Arterial oxygen saturation during nasotracheal suctioning. Chest 76:283, 1979
107. Kerem E, Yatsiv I, Goiten K: The effects of endotracheal suctioning on arterial blood gas in children. Intensive Care Med 16:95, 1990
108. Boutros A: Arterial blood oxygenation during and after endotracheal suctioning in the apneic patient. Anesthesiology 32:114, 1970
109. Walsh J, Van der Warf C, Hoscheit D: Unsuspected hemodynamic alterations during endotracheal suctioning. Chest 95:162, 1989
110. Kelly R, Yao F, Artusio J: Prevention of suction-induced hypoxemia by simultaneous oxygen insufflation. Crit Care Med 15: 874, 1987
111. Berman I, Stahl W: Prevention of hypoxic complication during endotracheal suctioning. Surgery 63:586, 1968
112. Taylor P, Waters H: Arterial oxygen tensions following endotracheal suctioning on IPPV. Anaesthesia 26:289, 1971
113. Winston S, Gravelyn T, Sitrin R: Prevention of bradycardiac responses to endotracheal suctioning by prior administration of nebulized atropine. Crit Care Med 15:1,009, 1987
114. Frankel H, Mathias C, Spalding J: Mechanisms of reflex cardiac arrest in tetraplegic patients. Lancet 2: 1,183, 1975
115. Clark A, Winslow E, Tyler D et al: The effects of endotracheal suctioning on mixed venous oxygen saturation and heart rate in critically ill adults. Heart Lung 19:552, 1990
116. Durand M, Sangha B, Cabal L et al: Cardipulmonary and intracranial pressure changes related to endotracheal suctioning in preterm infants. Crit Care Med. 17:506, 1989
117. Fanconi S, Duc G: Intratracheal suctioning in sick preterm infants: prevention of intracranial hypertension and cerebral hypoperfusion by muscle paralysis. Pediatrics 79:538, 1987
118. Rosen M, Hillard E: The effects of negative pressure during tracheal suction. Anesth Analg 41:50, 1962
119. Demers R, Saklad M: The etiology, pathophysiology and treatment of atelectasis. Respir Care: 21:234, 1976
120. Demers R: Complications of endotracheal suctioning procedures. Respir Care 27:453, 1982
121. Kleiber C, Krutzfield N, Rose E: Acute histologic changes in the tracheobronchial tree associated with different suction catheter insertion techniques. Heart Lung 17:10, 1988
122. Brodsky L, Reidy M, Stanievich J: The effects of suctioning techniques on the distal tracheal mucosa in intubated low birth weight infants. Int J Pediatr Otorhinolaryngol 14:1, 1987
123. Kuzenski B: Effect of negative pressure in tracheobronchial trauma. Nurs Res 27:260, 1978
124. Jung R, Gottleib L: Comparison of tracheobronchial suction catheters in humans. Chest 69:179, 1967
125. Deppe S, Kelly J, Thoi L: Incidence of colonization, nosocomial pneumonia, and mortality in critically ill patients using trach care closed suction system versus an open suction system: prospective randomized study. Crit Care Med 18:1,389, 1990
126. Rindfleisch S, Typer M: The effects of duration of endotracheal suctioning on arterial oxygenation in anaesthetized dogs, abstracted, part 2. Am Rev Respir Dis 123:19, 1981

127. Chulay M: arterial blood gas changes with a hyperinflation and hyperoxygenation suctioning intervention in critically ill patients. Heart Lung 17:654, 1988

128. Gold M, Duarte I, Muravchick S: Arterial oxygenation in conscious patients after 5 minutes and after 30 seconds of oxygen breathing. Anesth Analg 60:313, 1981

129. Preusser B, Stone S, Gonyon D et al: Effects of two methods of preoxygenation on mean arterial pressure, cardiac output, peak airway pressure and post suctioning hypoxemia. Heart Lung 17:290, 1988

130. Chulay M: Efficacy of a hyperinflation and hyperoxygenation suctioning intervention. Heart Lung 17:15, 1988

131. Rogge J, Bunde L, Baun M: Effectiveness of oxygen concentrations of less than 100% before and after endotracheal suction in patients with chronic obstructive pulmonary disease. Heart Lung 18:64, 1989

132. Brown S, Stanbury D, Merell E et al: Prevention of suction-related arterial oxygen desaturation: comparison of off-ventilatror and on-ventilatior suctioning. Chest 83:621, 1983

133. DeCampo T, Civetta J: The effect of short term discontinuation of high level PEEP in patients with acute respiratory failure. Crit Care Med 7:47, 1979

134. Kumar A, Falke K, Giffin B et al: Continuous positive pressure ventilation in acute respiratory failure: effects on hemodynamics and lung function. N Engl J Med 283:1,430, 1970

135. Noll M, Hix C, Scott G: Closed tracheal suction systems: effectiveness and nursing implications. AACN Clin Issues Crit Care Nurs 1:318, 1990

136. Carlon G, Fox S, Ackerman N: Evaluation of a closed-tracheal suction system. Crit Care Med 15:522, 1987

137. Bodai B: A means of suctioning without cardiopulmonary depression. Heart Lung 11:172, 1982

138. Belling D, Kelley R, Simon R: Use of the swivel adaptor during suctioning to prevent hypoxemia in the mechanically ventilated patient. Heart Lung 7:320, 1978

139. Cabal L, Devaskar S, Siassi B et al: New endotracheal tube adaptor reducing cardiopulmonary effects of suctioning. Crit Care Med 7:552, 1979

140. Taggart J, Dorinsky N, Sheahan J: Airway pressures during closed system suctioning. Heart Lung 15:536, 1988

141. Stone K: Ventilator versus manual resuscitation bag as the method for delivering hyperoxygenation before endotracheal suctioning. AACN Clin Issues Crit Care Nurs 1:289, 1990

142. Benson M, Pierson D: Ventilator wash out volume: a consideration in endotracheal suction preoxygenation. Respir Care 24:832, 1979

143. Bien M, Liao S, Wang J: The function of 100% O_2 suction key in Bennett 7200 Microprocessor Ventilator, abstracted. Chung Hua I Hsueh Tsa Chih 45:39, 1990

144. Hanley M, Rudd T, Butler J: What happens to intratracheal saline instillations? Am Rev Resp Dis 117:124, 1978

145. Ackerman M: The use of bolus normal saline instillations in artificial airways: is it useful or necessary? Heart Lung 14:505, 1985

146. Bodai B, Walton C, Briggs S et al: A clinical evaluation of an oxygen insufflation/ suction catheter. Heart Lung 16:39, 1987

147. Spoerel W, Chan C: Jet ventilation for tracheobronchial suctioning. Anesthesiology 45:450, 1976

148. Guntupalli K, Sladen A, Klain M: High frequency jet ventilation (HFJV) in the prevention of a decrease in PaO_2 during suctioning, abstracted. Chest 80:381, 1981

149. Bostick J, Wendelgass S: Normal saline instillation as part of the suctioning procedure: effects on PaO_2 and amount of secretions. Heart Lung 16:532, 1987

7 | Breathing Exercises

Claudia R. Levenson

Breathing exercises have long been used by practitioners with widely varying goals. The objectives or desired outcomes have ranged from relaxation and pain control as is seen in transcendental meditation, evoking the relaxation response for stress reduction, to pain control as seen in natural childbirth, using breathing patterns. Most commonly, breathing exercises and patterns are employed to increase lung volume and improve gas exchange in the treatment of lung pathology.

Strength and endurance training exercises of the ventilatory muscles involve another form of breathing exercise used predominantly to improve pulmonary function and increase exercise capacity. The purposeful alteration of a given breathing pattern is also considered among the therapeutic interventions commonly categorized as breathing exercises. Each form of breathing exercise described can be used alone or in combination with other techniques to improve gas exchange and increase the mechanical advantage of the ventilatory pump. The goal of these exercises is to decrease or prevent pulmonary impairment and increase physical functional capacity. However, the use of breathing exercises has not been within the exclusive domain of medical practice.

The religious use of breathing exercises was described extensively in 1958 by Ha'Nish,[1] in a guide to the Mazdaznan culture and teachings, which rely heavily on the use of breathing exercises in combination with prayer. In an introductory lesson, Ha'Nish describes how prayer is "uttered on the breath, i.e., on one single exhalation, to assure oxygenation, purification of the blood, increased circulation, and rhythmic heart action".[1] The breathing exercise advocated can be identified as a sustained maximal inspiration followed by prolonged active expiration through pursed lips as the prayer is completed. The claim of improved oxygenation, blood purification (removal of CO_2), increased circulation, and rhythmic heart action (improved [$\dot{V}_A : \dot{Q}$] matching and increased venous return) may very well have physiologic credibility.

Much of the confusion regarding the clinical use of breathing exercises, patterns, or strategies is due to lack of clarity in terminology. Most familiar are the terms relaxation breathing exercises, diaphragmatic breathing exercise, or better yet, relaxation diaphragmatic breathing exercises. As research has clarified the physiologic components of the breathing pattern and more accurately described the ventilatory muscles, the armamentarium of breathing exercises and nomenclature has expanded to include

> sustained maximal inspiration (SMI)
> pursed lip breathing (PLB)
> breathing retraining (BRT)
> ventilatory or respiratory muscle training (VMT or RMT)

This chapter therefore uses operational definitions to describe and discuss each breathing technique, its physiologic basis, and some possible methods for implementation. Exercise goals incorporate the physiologic and pathophysiologic principles described in Chapters 2 and 3 and are directed at reducing impairment and improving physical function.

BREATHING EXERCISES TO INCREASE LUNG VOLUME, REDISTRIBUTE VENTILATION, AND IMPROVE GAS EXCHANGE

In 1915 MacMahon[2] described the problems of lung collapse and dyspnea in the postsurgical patient. The physiologic problems associated with collapse were addressed therapeutically with specifically designed simple deep breathing exercises. Despite over 70 years of research regarding the anatomy and physiology of ventilatory muscles, physiology of ventilation, and the pathophysiology and the kinesiopathology of the pulmonary system, many of the simplest concepts have held true over time. Breathing exercises to increase lung volume, redistribute ventilation, and improve gas exchange are still commonly used and effective.

Physiologic Basis

General physiologic consequences of acute and chronic processes that produce atelectasis, collapse, and reduced lung volume include

1. Increased risk of infection secondary to impaired phagocytic action of alveolar macrophages in collapsed areas
2. Decreased neutrophil motility in patients undergoing or receiving general anesthesia[3,4,5]
3. Impaired gas exchange due to loss of surface area, causing hypoxemia, hypercarbia, dyspnea, and eventually, if untreated, acute respiratory failure
4. Potential for prolonged hospitalization with resultant deconditioning and loss of functional mobility

Table 3-2 illustrates the potential physiologic compromise that can occur with specific pathologic conditions and pulmonary impairments. The breathing exercises discussed in this section are those that are useful for treating the following categories of impairment (see Table 7-1):

1. Decreased intrathoracic–lung volume, atelectasis
2. Decreased chest wall–lung compliance
3. Increased flow resistance as a result of decreased lung volume
4. $\dot{V}_A : \dot{Q}$ mismatch

Techniques

Breathing exercise techniques include (see Table 7-2):

1. SMI (with and without use of incentive spirometers)
2. Diaphragmatic breathing exercises
3. Segmental breathing exercises

Increasing lung volume in subjects with pain and mechanical disadvantage requires the direct attention of the therapist and subject. Pain control through medication and positioning may improve mechanics and gain cooperation of the patient. Techniques of proprioceptive neuromuscular facilitation (PNF) and chest wall mobilization (stretch, resistance, etc.) are commonly used to facilitate patient control and cooperation with the exercise. Airway clearance tech-

Table 7-1. Breathing Exercises/Strategies to Reduce or Correct Physiologic Compromise

Physiologic Compromise	Breathing Exercise/Strategy
Group I	
Decreased intrathoracic–lung volume	Sustained maximal inspiratory maneuvers
Decreased chest wall–lung compliance	(SMI)
Increased flow resistance resulting from	Diaphragmatic breathing exercises
decreased lung volume	Segmental breathing exercises
$\dot{V}_A : \dot{Q}$ mismatch	
Group II	
Decreased lung–thorax compliance	Strength/endurance training
Decreased intrathoracic volume in	Inspiratory resistance training (IMT)
neuromuscular or musculoskeletal	Isocapneic hyperpnea
impairments	
Increased flow resistance/airway obstruction	
Change in length/tension/force generation	
Group III	
Increased work (elastic and flow resistive)	Diaphragmatic breathing exercises
Decreased compliance/increased resistance/	Pursed lip breathing (PLB)
load work; diaphragm/accessories	Paced breathing with exercise (PBE)
Change in length/tension/force generation	Exhale with exercise/activity (EWE)
mechanical disadvantage	
$\dot{V}_A : \dot{Q}$ mismatch	

Table 7-2. Breathing Exercise Techniques

Technique	Explanation
Sustained maximal inspiration (SMI)	Maximal inspiratory effort slowly inhaled through nose to total lung capacity—3 sec hold at maximum inspiration
Diaphragmatic breathing exercises	Incorporation of body position with tactile and verbal cueing and resistance to improve diaphragmatic recruitment/excursion during inspiration/expiration
Segmental breathing exercises	Incorporation of positioning with tactile and verbal cueing and resistance to enhance localized expansion of a specific lung segment to facilitate chest wall motion and increase ventilation

niques described in Chapters 5 and 6 can be performed with these exercises as part of a bronchopulmonary hygiene or airway clearance treatment. The literature investigating successful use of these exercises is difficult to interpret as related to the breathing exercises alone. Most studies describe the collective use of a series of techniques. Consequently, specific descriptions are included here whenever possible and related to the literature as it is currently possible.

All three breathing exercise techniques (SMI, diaphragmatic, and segmental) are designed to increase intrathoracic lung volume. This is accomplished by taking advantage of the intrinsic muscle properties of length–tension and force velocity. Any stimulation to the skeletal ventilatory muscles can increase the contraction force generated during inspiration and produce added chest wall displacement, thereby decreasing intrathoracic pressure and increasing gas flow and lung volume. The breathing exercise is designed to take advantage of the musculoskeletal pump's construction and intrinsic properties to facilitate gas flow:

1. Inspiration is *slow* to decrease velocity and increase strength of muscle contraction. Flow occurs preferably through the nose to provide adequate resistance but may also occur through pursed lips.

2. Maximum inspiration is prolonged, with the volume sustained at end inspiration to encourage recruitment of all possible muscle fibers and to achieve the greatest drop in intrathoracic pressure, thereby enhancing distribution of gas with high inspiratory volume.[6]

3. Inspiratory muscle contraction force is maximized with tactile input in the form of stretch before inspiration, and resistance is applied throughout to take advantage of the muscle's optimum length–tension relationship.

4. Intrathoracic–lung volume is further enhanced by incorporating patterns of motion that recruit inspiratory musculature and encourage chest wall elevation and expansion, that is, bilateral upper extremity flexion and external rotation or unilateral upper extremity flexion/abduction/external rotation patterns.

5. Exhalation in this setting is passive.

Implementation

The goals of these breathing exercises are to increase inhaled volume, sustain alveolar inflation, and maintain or restore functional residual capacity (FRC).[6–8] These breathing exercises are generally used for the surgical population, subjects with chest wall pain or loss of mobility and restrictive disorders. An SMI maneuver is a common treatment choice in acute situations (e.g., post-trauma, postsurgery, or in the treatment of acute lobar collapse). Its positive effect in the postoperative population has been reviewed extensively.[6,9,10,11] Continued controversy about the best method to attain hourly SMI has fueled many discussions. Agreement centers around timing (hourly), a negative pressure inspiration being most effective, and a prolonged hold at maximum inspiration.[6,7,9]

Diaphragmatic and segmental breathing have been purported to achieve other physiologic effects, depending on the method of instruction and the individual being trained.[12–16] Roussos and Fixley et al.[12] were able to demonstrate differences in the distribution of inhaled gas during spontaneous versus intercostal versus abdominal augmented breathing patterns in varying positions with normal subjects. Specific segmental gas distribution has not been demonstrated to be possible in COPD patients regardless of position or breathing pattern employed.[12,13,14] However, it is highly possible that the physiologic benefit of diaphragmatic breathing for COPD patients lies not in the specific redistribution of inspired gas, but in improved overall gas distribution at higher lung volumes and a decreased energy cost of ventilation due to a more efficient, slower, deeper respiratory pattern.[13–16] This concept is explained further in the last section of this chapter, in the discussion of strategies for breathing.

In addition to the commonly cited causative factors of pain (direct injury, monotonous ventilatory pattern, and inactivity that contribute to lung collapse), diaphragmatic dysfunction has also been thought to play a significant role in postoperative pulmonary dysfunction.[8,17–19] The contribution has been particularly suspect in upper abdominal surgeries. Studies examining efficacy of various treatment techniques or breathing exercises used in the postoperative population have had varied results, perhaps because of the varying degrees of diaphragmatic dysfunction believed to occur with different surgeries.[19,20–22]

The mechanism of diaphragmatic dysfunction appears to be reflex mediated by stimulation of visceral or somatic efferent pathways during surgery, causing inhibition of phrenic nerve output.[18,23] Chuter et al. demonstrated in 1988 that routine incentive spirometry did not improve the diaphragmatic dysfunction found in eight postcholecystectomy women.[19] Voluntary diaphragmatic movement is thought to be preserved postoperatively.[18] Positioning and breathing exercises that encourage increased activation or recruitment of the diaphragm, in addition to those that enhance the chest wall excursion, should probably be used; they are common in physical therapy treatment sessions. Vraciu and Vraciu successfully employed positioning and deep breathing exercises to significantly reduce post-operative complications in a group of thoracic surgical patients.[21] Although potentially success could be attributed to lack of diaphragmatic dysfunction, a comparison control group had a complication rate similar to that seen in untreated postoperative abdominal surgical patients.[21,22]

Adoption of breathing exercise techniques to increase lung/thoracic volume will most likely be successful in the setting where there is no neuromuscular or musculoskeletal impairment causing similar physiologic compromise (see Table 3-2). Appropriate or additional techniques to enhance performance for subjects with these neuromusculoskeletal impairments are discussed in the following section.

BREATHING EXERCISES TO INCREASE STRENGTH, ENDURANCE, AND EFFICIENCY

The muscles that comprise the ventilatory pump perform the elastic and flow resistive work of breathing (WOB) day in and day out. The capacity of the pump to perform this work is enormous (a maximum voluntary ventilation [MVV] of 200 L/min in world-class athletes) in the normal population and therefore rarely a limiting factor in exercise performance. This does not necessarily hold true for the population with respiratory impairment that decreases the ventilatory reserve capacity and increases the WOB.

Physiologic Basis

Physiologic consequences of decreased ventilatory muscle strength and/or endurance include

1. Decreased lung volume with resultant physiologic sequelae previously described (Group I–see Table 7-1)
2. Decreased cough effectiveness
3. Decreased maximum work capacity of the ventilatory pump in situations of increased oxygen demand (e.g., infection) or increased pump workload demand (e.g., exercise, ventilator weaning)
4. Decreased efficiency of the pump or increased O_2 cost of ventilation

Techniques

Treatment techniques to enhance the expulsive quality of the cough are discussed in Chapter 6. While positioning, neuromuscular facilitation, and mechanical stimulation are all valuable techniques, ventilatory muscle strength is an important factor in improving cough quality as well. Strength of the inspiratory muscles directly affects the inspired volume available to help generate high expiratory flow rates, and the expiratory muscles are crucial in generating adequate expiratory force. Techniques discussed in this section can also be used to improve cough strength.

Strength and/or endurance training techniques include ventilatory muscle training, inspiratory muscle training, inspiratory threshold loading, isocapneic hyperpnea, and respiratory muscle rest therapy (see Table 7-3), and are considered as a component of the patient's comprehensive program when pulmonary impairments (see Table 7-1) include

1. Decreased lung–thorax compliance
2. Decreased intrathoracic volume in the setting of neuromuscular or musculoskeletal compromise
3. Increased flow resistance/airway obstruction
4. Change in the length–tension relationship of ventilatory muscles

Implementation

Clinical measures (see Ch. 4) that aid in determining the degree of impairment and potential limitation also assist in documenting posttreatment improvement. There are many valid, reliable ways to measure the muscle strength and endurance of the ventilatory pump. However, only a few of these are clinically useful. To measure strength (intrathoracic pressure change elicited with maximum contraction against an obstructed airway), maximal inspiratory and expiratory pressures (MIP, MEP) are used. Vital capacity (VC) is an indicator of strength comparing actual total volume moved to a predicted value for the size

Table 7-3. Strength and/or Endurance Training Techniques

Technique	Explanation
Ventilatory muscle training (VMT)	Synonomous with respiratory muscle training. Encompasses all forms of strength and endurance training methods for the ventilatory muscles
Inspiratory muscle training (IMT)	Synonomous with inspiratory resistance loading. Resistive loads are applied during the inspiratory phase. If ventilation is maintained or increased, there is a volume as well as a resistance load placed on the ventilatory muscles. Endurance and strength training can then occur
Inspiratory threshold loading	Category of inspiratory muscle training: the use of weights or spring devices to determine opening pressure of a one-way valve during inspiration. As with other forms of IMT, breathing patterns can vary. If ventilation is maintained or increased, an endurance, as well as strength training, response can occur
Isocapneic hyperpnea	Synonomous with normocarbic hyperpnea: the use of a target ventilatory level under isocapneic conditions. This can simulate the volume load on the ventilatory muscles during exercise, producing primarily an endurance training effect
Respiratory muscle rest therapy (RMR)	Employment of any therapeutic device that performs a portion of all of the mechanical work of the ventilatory pump

and age of an individual. Measures of endurance (anything expressed as a repeated volume calculated per unit of time) include minute ventilation ($\dot{V}e$), MVV, and maximal sustainable ventilatory capacity (MSVC). A measure of efficiency would be the oxygen cost of a given level of ventilatory pump work (e.g., $\dot{V}e$). Once the presence of one or more pulmonary impairments has been identified, measurements are obtained to determine whether ventilatory muscle strength, endurance, or both are diminished.

In 1976, Leith and Bradley demonstrated that it was possible to train the ventilatory muscles of normal subjects for increases in strength and endurance.[24] Subjects trained to increase strength (MIP/MEP) using repeated maximum static inspiratory and expiratory maneuvers. Endurance trainers performed normocarbic hyperpnea as the training method to increase MSVC. Both groups trained for 30 to 45 minutes per day, 5 days per week. Strength trainers improved strength only, and endurance training improved endurance only. The fact that no cross-over occurred between strength and endurance trainers demonstrated that specificity of training probably applies to the skeletal ventilatory muscles, in addition to skeletal limb muscles.

Shortly after Leith and Bradley's study, additional literature appeared demonstrating similar increases in ventilatory muscle strength and endurance of subjects with pulmonary impairment (cystic fibrosis, chronic obstructive pulmonary disease [COPD], and muscular dystrophy).[25–27] Not surprisingly, study results differed among groups, as various methods were used for training and subjects differed in diagnosis and degree of impairment. Generally, methods that specifically trained the ventilatory muscles for an increase in strength or endurance were able to demonstrate improvement in those parameters. Studies that attempted to produce change in pulmonary function parameters or increased functional activity performance were not routinely successful.

Training devices were subsequently developed to assist patients perform a combination of ventilatory muscle strength and endurance training. Subjects were instructed to breathe at a preset rate and volume through a narrowed orifice, theoretically increasing resistance to inspiratory flow, and thereby loading the muscles for time periods usually in the 15- to 30-minute range. The training modality was labeled "inspiratory resistance loading" (synonymous with inspiratory muscle training [IMT]), and in controlled situations, produced changes in both strength and endurance.[26,28] Controls included ensuring that subjects moved a predetermined volume at a predetermined rate. Without such controls, subjects were found to decrease rate and volume during training runs, thereby reducing ventilatory load.

Inspiratory loading is the most common form of ventilatory muscle training (VMT) used in clinical practice today, despite unanswered questions regarding the usefulness of improved strength and endurance of the ventilatory muscles. Many clinicians ask if IMT improves exercise tolerance. If IMT improves exercise performance, in what populations and under what clinical conditions does change occur? What is the best method for training? Where does IMT fit in the treatment regimen? If patients simply perform functional activities, will this preclude the need for IMT, or are the benefits additional?

In 1980, Belman and Mittman used isocapneic hyperpnea as a training method with 10 COPD patients and were able to demonstrate improvement in exercise performance in addition to increased ventilatory muscle endurance and efficiency.[29] Their findings of improved exercise performance were also found by investigators using IMT[30] and were not reproducible by others.[28,31,32] Interestingly, when these studies are more closely compared (Table 7-4), it appears that in addition to differences in training methods and outcomes measured, the level of disability at initiation of training had a marked effect on the subject's degree of benefit from any form of therapy.[28,30] Potentially, subjects with significant impairment will respond to a variety of therapeutic interventions, while healthier subjects may require more specific programs directed at individual impairments.

In 1982, Belman and Kendregan took a slightly different approach and studied whether exercise training with arm or leg ergometry without breathing

Table 7-4. Results of Ventilatory Muscle Training

Author	Population	Method	Results
Belman[29]	10 COPD patients	6 weeks: twice daily 15-minute MSVC training runs	No change in lung volume or flow. Increased MSVC, maximum exercise ventilation during exercise test, and 12-minute walking distance
Chen[31]	13 COPD patients (6, control; 7, IMT)	Controls used sham IMT. IMT trained with resistive load. Twice daily 15 min for 4 weeks	No change in controls. IMT group increased sustainable inspiratory pressure. No change in PFTs or exercise capacity
Pardy[30]	17 COPD patients (9, control; 8, IMT)	Controls exercised for 4 weeks. No standard intensity or duration. IMT group performed inspiratory resistance training 30 minutes daily	Controls increase 12-minute walk distance. IMT increased 12-minute walking distance and endurance time on IMT
Pardy[30]	12 patients with moderate to severe COPD	Inspiration against critical resistance for 15-minute sessions twice daily. Retest at 1 and 2 months	Increased muscle endurance. No change in strength. Seven patients increased exercise test endurance time
Belman[33]	15 COPD patients (8, arm trainers; 7, leg trainers)	20-minute arm/leg ergometry for 6 weeks	No change in lung volume or flow. Increase in mean endurance workload for 20 minutes on arm or leg. No change in MSVC

Abbreviations: COPD, chronic obstructive pulmonary disease; IMT, inspiratory muscle training; PFT, pulmonary function test; MSVC, maximal sustainable ventilatory capacity.

training would in turn improve ventilatory muscle performance.[33] They could not demonstrate any change in MSVC or PFTs in the training group, which again raises the question of what form of training is most useful. The subjects involved did improve lower extremity strength and endurance, which may have been functionally more significant for that population.

Once decreased strength and endurance of ventilatory muscles has been documented, indicating training would be of added benefit, the best method and piece of equipment are selected. As stated previously, the most commonly used training method is some form of inspiratory resistive loading. Training devices usually consist of a mouthpiece attached to a one-way valve and a selection of progressively narrowed orifices that can be placed in the inspiratory port. Most include a second port for oxygen delivery if necessary (see Fig. 7-1).

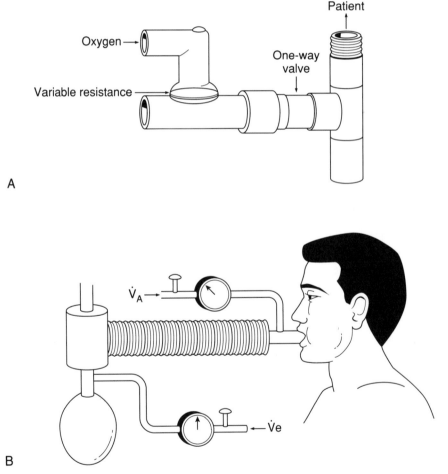

Fig. 7-1. (**A & B**) Training devices for increasing strength and endurance of ventilatory muscles. ($\dot{V}_A$, alveolar ventilation; $\dot{V}_e$, ventilation). (Fig. A adapted from Aldrich and Karpel,[35] with permission. Fig. B adapted from Leith and Bradley,[24] with permission.)

Many training methods have been proposed, but exercise prescription with these devices is recommended as follows:

1. Measure MIP.
2. Use measured MIP to calculate training load at 30 to 40 percent of the patient's maximum pressure.
3. Begin training exercise with the load (orifice, setting) that elicits the 30 to 40 percent level of maximum inspiratory pressure.
4. Have the patient breathe against that pressure at resting respiratory rate and tidal volume for up to 15 minutes if possible.
5. Training periods should total 30 minutes daily.
6. If the patient is unable to sustain 15 minutes continuously, interval training can be done initially (e.g., 5- or 10-minute segments), leading to a goal of 15 to 30 minutes of continuous exercise.

There are inherent problems with this procedure and these devices:

1. The less expensive devices most commonly do not allow for simple monitoring or regulation of inspiratory pressure during use.
2. There is no mechanism for control of RR, Vt or flow rate.
3. Patients not only choose their own respiratory pattern, but often slow their respiratory rate and decrease their volume/flow to reduce the workload. As these changes occur unmonitored, the patient will appear to be making progress (achieving 30 minutes of training) and be directed to proceed to a greater load (narrower orifice), while still functioning at the initial level. These subjects may achieve no benefit at all. These problems with control may account for some of the discrepancies in results among various researchers. An even worse case scenario occurs in the patient who chooses to reduce the workload, under-ventilates, and becomes hypercarbic in the process.[34]

There are two possible solutions to this dilemma. Initially the patient is given a predetermined target minute ventilation at which to train. Compliance can then most simply be monitored by attaching a spirometer in the inspiratory limb to record volume and using a metronome to count rate. If there is concern about adequacy of gas exchange with a particular patient, noninvasive monitoring of oxygen saturation/pressure of end tidal carbon dioxide (SaO_2/$PetCO_2$) may be required. I have found this to be necessary only in the ICU setting.

An alternative threshold training device has more recently become commercially available (Threshold IMT, Healthscan). The device includes a mouthpiece attached to a spring-loaded one-way valve that opens to permit airflow once the preset inspiratory pressure has been achieved. With the use of this device, there is better assurance of a minimum workload being maintained and better chance for successful strength and endurance training. The previously outlined procedure can be followed to set load. Again, the breathing strategy is not controlled, so the volume load will differ between patients, as will the training effect. Since the workload or pressure is consistent with this device, it is in effect more difficult, and most patients must begin at the lowest setting. They are progressed when they can perform at the current setting for 15 to 20 minutes continuously. The therapist and patient must be aware that detraining occurs once training has ceased, as it does with other skeletal muscles.

Treatment of patients with ventilatory muscle weakness and inability to wean from mechanical ventilation are likely candidates for this form of treatment. In 1985, Aldrich and Karpel used inspiratory resistance training with four patients previously unable to wean.[35] Three of the four patients experienced an increase in inspiratory muscle strength, VC, and tolerance to t-piece trials. Literature surrounding the use of VMT in this population is limited.

In the case of chronic or acute respiratory failure, ventilatory muscle fatigue potentially plays a role. Instinctually, the therapist might consider further loading of the muscles with VMT to improve strength and endurance, as in the case of Aldrich and Karpel.[35] On the other hand, when dealing with muscles that are already fatiguing, it may be prudent to incorporate some form of respiratory muscle rest therapy (RMR). Techniques discussed in previous chapters, such as drug therapy and airway clearance techniques, decrease the WOB or ventilatory pump demand and could be thought of as forms of rest therapy.[36] RMR is usually considered as an additional therapy in the form of intermittent negative or positive pressure ventilation and can be another method for improving ventilatory muscle strength and endurance.

In 1983, Rabinovitch et al. described the use of negative pressure for 1 hour to rest the muscles of COPD patients.[37] This rest period produced measureable increases in transdiaphragmatic pressure. Cropp and Dimarco used a similar method of negative pressure ventilation with COPD patients intermittently over three days to rest the ventilatory muscles.[38] Their subjects showed significantly elevated strength values and lowered partial arterial pressure of carbon dioxide ($PaCO_2$) when compared to a similar control group during the same time period. Braun and Marino also reported significant improvements (increased VC, MVV, maximal inspiratory pressure [PI max], maximal expiratory pressure [PE max], and decreased $PaCO_2$) in subjects with chronic respiratory failure who used negative or positive assist ventilation nightly for 6 months.[39] Other investigators using similar methods have not been as successful in demonstrating the same positive results from RMR therapy.[40,41] Levine[36] gives a detailed description of the literature surrounding this subject. Much discussion and research still needs to be done to determine the appropriate roles of exercise conditioning, VMT, and RMR in the treatment of patients in chronic respiratory failure.

BREATHING STRATEGIES TO DECREASE WORK OF BREATHING AND SENSATION OF DYSPNEA AND TO IMPROVE VENTILATION EFFICIENCY

Physiologic Basis

The first two sections of this chapter examined techniques to maximize gas exchange and/or improve ventilatory pump strength/endurance. These treatments or methods of training are employed to effect change over a course of treatment and time with specific goals in mind. This last section deals with breathing strategies for patients with chronic pulmonary impairment (see Group III, Table 7-1). These are strategies that patients might additionally learn and use during training. They may also use such strategies in everyday life to assist them with symptoms of dyspnea to decrease pulmonary limitations to activities of daily living (ADL). Consequently, they are labeled strategies, rather than exercises. Patients generally find these extremely useful if they are easily learned. Symptomatic complaints indicating that potential benefit may be gained from use of these techniques are

1. Complaints of dyspnea at rest or with minimal activity
2. Inability to perform ADLs due to pulmonary limitation
3. Use of inefficient breathing patterns during ADLs or exercise training

The physiologic consequences of pulmonary impairment that may be positively impacted by these strategies include increased elastic and flow resistive work of breathing, mechanical disadvantage of ventilatory muscles (length–tension, force–velocity), and $\dot{V}_A\dot{Q}$ mismatch.

Techniques

Breathing strategies (Table 7-5) include

1. Diaphragmatic breathing exercises
2. Pursed lip breathing (PLB)
3. Paced breathing with exercise (PBE)
4. Exhale with exercise/activity (EWE)

These are the techniques that most commonly come under the heading of breathing retraining (BRT). When the oxygen demand increases in normal individuals and $\dot{V}e$ must increase in response, the enormous reserve capacity of the ventilatory pump allows this to occur with relative ease and at minimum oxygen cost. Chapter 3 describes in detail the impact of pulmonary pathology on reserve capacity. When the impaired patient attempts to increase $\dot{V}e$, there may be a limited resource to draw upon and work may be accomplished at an enormous oxygen cost. All of the strategies listed here attempt to decrease the mechanical disadvantage of the impaired ventilatory pump and thereby decrease the WOB to concomitantly decrease oxygen cost.

Implementation

Diaphragmatic breathing has been described earlier in connection with a sustained maximal inspiratory maneuver as a method of increasing lung volume. This technique has not been found useful in specific distribution of gas flow in abnormals. However, it has been shown to be beneficial in controlling respira-

Table 7-5. Breathing Strategies

Strategy	Explanation
Breathing retraining (BRT)	Can encompass the use of all techniques/devices that alter a patient's current breathing pattern. This includes all types of breathing exercises defined in Tables 7-2 and 7-3, but is usually used in reference to those breathing exercises/strategies that alter the breath-to-breath tidal volume/rate in an effort to reduce oxygen consumption/work of breathing
Diaphragmatic breathing exercises	The incorporation of body position with tactile and verbal cueing and resistance to improve diaphragmatic recruitment/excursion during inspiration/expiration
Pursed lip breathing exercises (PLB)	The expiratory phase of the breathing cycle is done through the patient's pursed lips. The expiratory phase is usually passive, but a component of active expiration can be employed in certain instances
Paced breathing with exercise (PBE)	Encompasses low-frequency breathing techniques, but may refer to any change in respiratory rhythm or rate aimed at reducing dyspnea
Exhale with exercise/activity (EWE)	Used during activity/low-level exercise. Body motion occurs only during the expiratory phase of the respiratory cycle. Can be used alone or in conjunction with the above-listed techniques

tory rate and improving gas mixing in COPD patients.[42–44] Effective use of it as a breathing strategy includes incorporating facilitation techniques of stretch and resistance to enhance the length/tension/force generation of the diaphragm. The technique is performed as follows:

1. Position the patient to relax the abdominal muscles and provide the possibility of visual as well as tactile facilitation and feedback (Fig. 7-2).
2. Inspiration is slow, through the nose or pursed lips.
3. Expiration is slow and controlled with active abdominal muscle contraction throughout expiration.
4. Additional hand pressure may be applied over the abdominals at end expiration to assist with expiration and give added resistance prior to the next inspiration. (see Fig. 7-2B)

It is the last two steps that potentially increase the length and curvature of the diaphragm at end expiration and therefore provide a stretch and stimulation to enhance contractile force at the beginning of the next inspiration. This stretch and muscle control facilitates increased Vt, decreased inspiratory flow rate, and decreased RR. Decreased velocity of muscle contraction increases strength of contraction, while stretch and resistance increase it. Decreasing rate reduces frequency of contraction, potentially postponing fatigue. These mechanical changes have been discussed as reducing the WOB and improving the mechanics of breathing. Once learned at rest, this pattern can be used during ambulation, stair climbing, or other activities.

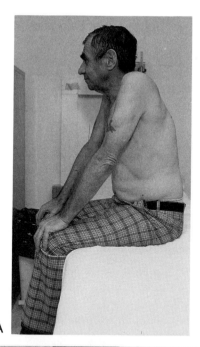

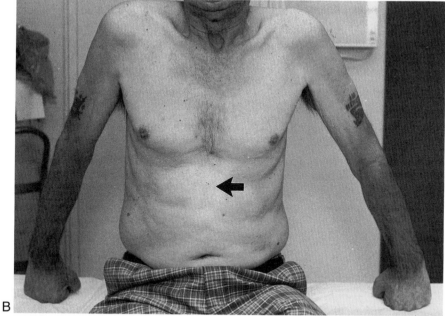

Fig. 7-2. Use of diaphragmatic breathing. (**A**) Seat the patient facing a mirror to observe his commonly assumed posture. Remove the arms from the stabilized position by flexing the elbows and externally rotating the arms. (**B**) Have the patient observe abdominal motion from face view and side view. Have the patient palpate abdominal contraction subcostally (arrow).

Patients' claims of relief of dyspnea and improved activity tolerance when incorporating this breathing strategy while performing ADLs have lead to many conflicting studies and reports regarding the benefits of the strategy. In 1954, Miller[15] reported improvements in Vt, VC, maximal breathing capacity, and gas exchange with use of controlled breathing patterns, while others were unable to corroborate these findings.[45] In 1955, Sinclair documented changes in diaphragmatic excursion with COPD subjects using a controlled diaphragmatic pattern, but no change in oxygen saturation was seen.[46] Interestingly enough, he did point out that subjects experienced a decrease in spinal and shoulder girdle motion during the controlled period. He postulated that a possible benefit of diaphragmatic breathing was the elimination of associated inefficient and costly muscle contraction. This has been suggested as another mechanism of improved efficiency and contribution to the benefit of diaphragmatic breathing.

Campbell and Friend[16] also investigated controlled diaphragmatic breathing and demonstrated no change in gas distribution or "mixing efficiency"; however, their subjects did show an increase in Vt and a decrease in RR. Sinclair attributed the subjective benefits associated with the technique to the actual change in breathing pattern, as had Campbell. In 1977, Brach et al., using radioactive xenon washout, again showed the inability to change the distribution of inspired gas using an augmented diaphragmatic breathing pattern.[13] Both normals and COPD subjects participated in the study and, although no preferential distribution of gas occurred, overall xenon washout improved during the controlled pattern time period. The authors again suggested that the improved gas exchange was due to a slower, deeper breathing pattern. Studies by Wade and others more definitely demonstrate that it is not possible to reliably measure improved gas distribution by observation of diaphragmatic movement.[47,48] Nor can change in lung volume be assumed from observing abdominal wall motion or changes in thoracoabdominal shape. Perhaps the best clinically observable parameter for judging the success or usefulness of diaphragmatic breathing is to assess for a slowly decreasing RR and subjective improvement of dyspnea.

Pursed lip breathing (PLB) is a breathing pattern/strategy adopted spontaneously by some patients. Because of their claims of dyspnea relief, it is taught to many others. PLB has been investigated because, like diaphragmatic breathing, while patients claim beneficial effects, the physiologic reason for relief is not completely understood.[49,50] Procedures for teaching PLB usually begin in a similar fashion to those for diaphragmatic breathing:

1. Patient inhales slowly through the nose or pursed lips.
2. Patient is instructed to purse lips prior to expiration.
3. Patient then exhales slowly, having been instructed to relax throughout exhalation.
4. Patient stops exhaling once exhalation of additional inspired volume is completed.
5. As the patient improves, the tactile and verbal cues are removed.

Patients who spontaneously perform PLB often demonstrate abdominal muscle contraction during expiration. This may produce the mechanical advantage described during diaphragmatic breathing and is therefore sometimes incorporated in PLB instructions. If this component is added, it is done with careful attention to not forcing expiration, which would cause increased airway collapse.

Many studies published during and after the 1960s attributed the benefits of PLB to increased Vt, decreased RR, and improved alveolar ventilation (increased efficiency of breathing), while others attributed benefits to the decrease in peak and mean expiratory flow rates (decreased WOB).[50–52] In 1970, Mueller et al. corroborated the occurrence of increased Vt and decreased RR with PLB.[49] Additionally, they found that the volume and rate change occurred during exercise as well as at rest, but the effects of improved oxygenation and alveolar ventilation only occurred at rest. Still another study, by Casciari et al., demonstrated improvement in exercise tolerance in severe COPD patients when BRT (composed of PLB with expiratory abdominal augmentation and accessory muscle use discouragement) was added to a regimen of exercise conditioning with treadmill walking.[53] Furthermore, the increased exercise tolerance in the BRT group occurred with a decreased RR and without a fall in oxygenation. Although the precise physiologic process is not yet absolutely clear, it appears that PLB can increase Vt and reduce RR without a decrease in $\dot{V}e$, and may, in certain cases, improve oxygenation and alveolar ventilation.

Paced breathing with activity is another strategy utilized to decrease the WOB and relieve dyspnea during activity/exercise. Unlike diaphragmatic breathing and PLB, paced breathing has not been extensively studied. The reason for this becomes more apparent upon examination of the procedure for teaching paced breathing. Patients seem to derive the most benefit from this strategy if they have perfected the skills of diaphragmatic breathing and PLB, but this is not essential. The patient and therapist simply test different inspiratory to expiratory (I : E) ratios with various activities until they find the rate and pattern that lowers RR, relieves dyspnea, and possibly improves SaO_2. As stated previously, prior skill with diaphragmatic breathing and PLB may provide added benefit. Certain activities such as cycling and walking, lend themselves readily to these techniques. Activities like stair climbing are tougher for severely impaired patients and require great concentration. This technique allows patients to control their dyspnea and become less fearful of activity and exercises.

Synchronization of $\dot{V}e$ with activity is another form of paced breathing. The synchronization and breath control learned with swimming is one of the reasons swimming has been recommended as a form of exercise training for asthmatics. On the other hand, the energy cost of swimming is extremely high and more severely impaired patients may find it too difficult. Control of dyspnea usually entails learning one or more of the previously described techniques/strategies and is one of several reasons that pulmonary-impaired patients do not do well with a wide variety of activities. For example, circuit training programs often include high oxygen–demand upper extremity activity and frequent change in activity that requires incorporating a variety of breathing patterns. Normal individuals tend to choose their breathing patterns according to the Vt and breathing frequency (fb) that is most mechanically efficient, but synchronization also influences this pattern during certain activities.[54]

As mentioned previously, COPD patients have a very limited capacity for increasing $\dot{V}e$ with exercise. Since they are often exhaling on the outer limits of their maximal flow volume curves at rest, they often demonstrate a disproportionate increase in fb with minimal exercise.[55] There are few breathing strategies available to meet increased oxygen demand in individuals with such limitations. They can shorten inspiratory time and prolong expiratory time, but this requires an increase in inspiratory flow with a decrease in inspiratory time (T_i) in relation to the total respiratory cycle time (T_{tot}) $T_i : T_{tot}$ with less time for the muscles to develop force. Or, they can breathe at high lung volume to increase expiratory flow. This also increases the elastic WOB for muscles already at a disadvantage.[55] The previously mentioned strategies attempt to maximize the ventilatory capacity, but in disease a ventilatory limit will eventually be reached.

Finally, exhale with effort (EWE) is a breathing strategy usually employed only with the most severely impaired patients or those with the greatest complaints of dyspnea. The procedure for this technique is to teach the patient to break any activity (e.g., bending, lifting, getting out of bed) into one or more breaths:

1. Inhale during rest (using diaphragmatic breathing pattern).
2. Exhale through pursed lips during activity.
3. Repeat sequence, stopping motion during inspiration and continuing until activity is accomplished.

Patients claim immediate and dramatic relief with this technique. Little literature exists concerning this, but in some ways it makes physiologic sense. It incorporates the principles involved in diaphragmatic breathing, PLB, and paced breathing, while additionally decreasing the rate of activity to reduce the metabolic demand for severely impaired patients. Control of breathing with activity also allows use of all ventilatory musculature during the active phase of breathing (inspiration) and performance of other skeletal muscle activity while the ventilatory muscles relax (expiration).

Most of the strategies in this section have been discussed in terms of their use in the COPD population. This is not to say that they do not have some application in patients with restrictive disease as well. Understandably, however, other patient populations may have fewer strategies available to them than COPD patients. Given the severe volume reductions imposed by restrictive disease, breathing frequency is usually the only method available to increase $\dot{V}e$. Attempts to change the breathing pattern as previously described will meet with very limited success. In some instances where decreased intrathoracic volume is a result of neuromuscular rather than musculoskeletal disease, improvement of the length–tension relationship for the inspiratory muscles with position and mechanical devices may possibly put more of these strategies to use.

SUMMARY

Breathing exercises play an important role in the treatment of pulmonary patients. The literature has in some cases been able to verify the physiologic changes and/or benefit therapists hope to effect, but in many others, it has not. Much more study is required. It is important, however, to develop and base therapeutic interventions on the physiologic compromises that may or may not be present in a disease state rather than on the disease itself.

REFERENCES

1. Ha'Nish OZA: The Power of the Breath. Llewellyn Publications, Los Angeles, 1958
2. MacMahon C: Breathing and physical exercises for use in cases of wounds in the pleura, lung, and diaphragm. Lancet 2:769, 1915
3. Shennib H, Mulder DS, Chiu RLJ: The effects of pulmonary atelectasis and re-expansion on lung cellular immune defenses. Arch Surgery. 119:275–277, 1984
4. Serota AI, Meyer RD, Wilson SE, Edestein RH, Finegold SM: Legionaire's disease in the post operative patient. J Surg Res 30:417, 1981
5. Nunn JF, O'Morain C: Nitrous oxide decreases motility of human neutrophils in vitro. Anesthesiology 56:45, 1982
6. Bartlett RH, Crop P, Hanson EL, et al: The physiology of yawning and its application to post-operative care. Surg Forum 21:222, 1970
7. Bartlett RH, Gazzaniga AB, Geraghty TR: Respiratory maneuvers to prevent post-operative pulmonary complications: a critical review. JAMA 224:1,017, 1973
8. Bendixen HH, Bullwinkel B, Hedky-White, J, et al: Atelectasis and shunting during spontaneous ventilation in anesthetized patients. Anesthesiol 25:297, 1964
9. Bartlett RH, Gazzaniga AB, Geraghty TR: The yawn maneuver: prevention and treatment of post-operative pulmonary complications. Surg Forum 22:196, 1971
10. Ward RJ, et al: An evaluation of post-operative respiratory maneuvers. Surg Gynecol Obstet 123:51, 1966
11. Ravin MB: Value of deep breaths in reversing post-operative hypoxemia. NY State J Med 66:244, 1966
12. Roussos CS, Fixley M, Gedest J, et al: Voluntary factors influencing the distribution of inspired gas. Am Rev Respir Dis 116:457, 1977
13. Brach BB, Chao RP, Sgroi VL, et al: ^{133}Xenon washout patterns during diaphragmatic breathing: studies in normal subjects and patients with COPD. Chest 71:735, 1977
14. Grimby G, Oxhoj H, Bake B: Effects of abdominal breathing on distribution of ventilation in obstructive lung disease. Clin Sci Molec Med 148:193, 1975
15. Miller WP: A physiological evaluation of the effects of diaphragmatic breathing training in patients with chronic pulmonary emphysema. Am J Med 17:471, 1954

16. Campbell EM, Friend J: Action of breathing exercise in pulmonary emphysema. Lancet 1:325, 1955

17. Murray JF: Indications for mechanical aids to assist lung inflation in medical patients. Am Rev Respir Dis 122:121, 1983

18. Ford GT, Whitelaw WA, Rosenal TW, et al: Diaphragm function after upper abdominal surgery in humans. Amer Rev Respir Dis 127:431, 1983

19. Chuter TA, Weissman C, Starker PM, Gump FE: Effect of incentive spirometry on diaphragmatic function after surgery. Surgery 105:488, 1989

20. Dripps RD, Deming MVN: Post-operative atelectasis and pneumonia: diagnosis, etiology and management based upon 1,240 cases of upper abdominal surgery. Ann Surg. 124:94, 1946

21. Vraciu JK, Vraciu RA: Effectiveness of breathing exercises in preventing pulmonary complications following open heart surgery. Phys Ther 57:1,367, 1977

22. Thoren L: Post-operative pulmonary complications: observations on their prevention by means of physiotherapy. Acta Chir Scand 107:193, 1954

23. Ford GT, Riveout KS, Bozdeck LK et al: Inhibition of breathing arising from the gallbladder. Physiologist 26:A38, 1983

24. Leith DE, Bradley M: Ventilatory muscle strength and endurance training. J Appl Physiol 41:508, 1976

25. Keens TG, Krastins IR, Wannamaker EM et al: Ventilatory muscle endurance training in normal subjects and patients with cystic fibrosis. Am Rev Respir Dis 116:853, 1977

26. Anderson JB, Bragsted L, Kann T et al: Resistive breathing training in severe chronic obstructive pulmonary disease: a pilot study. Scand J Respir Dis 60:151, 1979

27. DiMarco AF, Kelling J, Sajovic M et al: Respiratory muscle training in muscular dystrophy. Clin Res 30:427A, 1982

28. Asher MI, Pardy RL, Coates AL et al: The effects of inspiratory muscle training in patients with cystic fibrosis. Am Rev Respir Dis 126:855, 1982

29. Belman MJ, Mittman C: Ventilatory muscle training improves exercise capacity in chronic obstructive pulmonary disease patients. Am Rev Respir Dis 121:273, 1980

30. Pardy RL, Rivington RN, Despas PJ et al: The effects of inspiratory muscle training on exercise performance in chronic airflow limitation. Am Rev Respir Dis 123:426, 1981

31. Chen HI, Dukes R, Martin BJ et al: Inspiratory muscle training in patients with chronic obstructive pulmonary disease. Am Rev Respir Dis 131:251, 1985

32. Pardy RL, Rivington RN, Despas PJ et al: Inspiratory muscle training compared with physical therapy in patients with chronic airflow limitation. Am Rev Respir Dis 123:421, 1981

33. Belman MJ, Kendregan BA: Physical training fails to improve ventilatory muscle endurance in patients with chronic obstructive pulmonary disease. Chest 81:440, 1982

34. Jederlinic P, Muspratt JA, Miller MJ: Inspiratory muscle training in clinical practice: physiologic conditioning or habituation to suffocation? Chest 86:870, 1984

35. Aldrich TK, Karpel JP: Inspiratory resistive training in respiratory failure. Am Rev Respir Dis 131:461, 1985

36. Levine S, Henson D, Levy S: Respiratory muscle rest therapy. Clin Chest Med 9:297, 1988

37. Rabinovitch B, Pardy RL, Hussain SA et al: The acute effects of rest on ventilatory muscle (VM) function in patients with severe chronic air flow limitation (CAL). Physiologist 26:21 (abstract), 1983

38. Cropp A, DiMarco AF: Effects of daily intermittent rest of pressure ventilation on respiratory muscle function in patients with severe chronic obstructive pulmonary disease. Am Rev Respir Dis 135:1,056, 1987

39. Braun NM, Marino WD: Effect of daily intermittent rest of respiratory muscles in patients with severe chronic airflow limitations (CAL). Chest 85:595, 1984

40. Pluto LA, Fahey PJ, Sorenson L et al: Effect of eight weeks of intermittent negative pressure ventilation on exercise parameters in patients with severe chronic obstructive lung disease. Am Rev Respir Dis 131 (abstract), 1985

41. Zibrak JD, Federman EC, Kwa SL et al: Effect of negative pressure ventilatory assistance on pulmonary function in severe COPD. Chest 89:515S (abstract), 1986

42. Pfeiffer V, Pfeiffer A: Breathing patterns and gas mixing. Phys Ther 44:331, 1964

43. Motely H: The effects of slow deep breathing and the blood gas exchange within emphysema. Am Rev Respir Dis 88:485, 1963

44. Paul G, Eldridge F, Mitchell J et al: Some effects of slowing respiration rate in chronic emphysema and bronchitis. J Appl Physiol 21:877, 1966

45. Becklake MR, McGregor M, Goldman HI et al: A study of the effects of physiotherapy in chronic hypertrophic emphysema using lung function tests. Dis Chest 26:180, 1954

46. Sinclair JD: The effects of breathing exercise in pulmonary emphysema. Thorax 10:246, 1955

47. Wade OL: Movement of thoracic cage and diaphragm in respiration. J Physiol 124:193, 1954

48. Grassino AE, Bake B, Martin RR et al: Voluntary changes of thoracoabdominal shape and regional lung volumes in humans. J Appl Physiol 39:997, 1975

49. Mueller RE, Petty TL, Filley GS et al: Ventilation and arterial blood gas changes induced by pursed lips breathing. J Appl Physiol 28:784, 1970

50. Ingram R, Schilder D: Effect of pursed lips expiration on the pulmonary pressure flow relationship in obstructive lung disease. Am Rev Respir Dis 96:381, 1967

51. Thoman RL, et al: The efficacy of pursed-lips breathing in patients with chronic obstructive pulmonary disease. Am Rev Respir Dis 93:100, 1966

52. Ingram RH, Schielder DP: Effect of pursed lips expiration on the pulmonary pressure flow relationship in obstructive lung disease. Am Rev Respir Dis 96:831, 1967

53. Casciari RJ, Fairshter RD, Harrison A et al: Effects of breathing retraining in patients with chronic obstructive pulmonary disease. Chest 79:393, 1981

54. Åstrand PO, Rodahl K: Textbook of Work Physiology Physiologic Basis for Exercise. McGraw-Hill, New York, 1977

55. Pardy RL, Hussain SA, Macklem PT: The ventilatory pump in exercise. Clin Chest Med 5:35–49, 1984

8 | Mobilization and Exercise Conditioning

Elizabeth Dean
Jocelyn Ross

The cardiopulmonary unit consists of the heart and lungs working synergistically and in series with the peripheral circulation to effect oxygen transport, hence, oxygenation of the tissues.[1-4] Oxygen transport is determined by the integrated function of four components: (1) optimal distribution of ventilation ($\dot{V}e$) to the alveoli, (2) diffusion of gases across the alveolar capillary membrane, (3) perfusion of the lungs, and (4) gas transport to the tissues.[5] Regulatory control at the neuronal, humoral, and local tissue levels ensures that this integrated system, involving the ventilatory and cardiac pumps and the pulmonary and systemic circulations, adapts promptly and appropriately to physical stressors.[6] Two physical stressors that significantly challenge oxygen transport from moment to moment are position changes and changes in activity level.[6-9] The ability to maintain oxygen transport by responding rapidly and appropriately to these two potentially adverse conditions is tantamount to life.

This chapter describes a physiologic framework for exercise prescription for the patient with compromised oxygen transport. While principles for prescribing exercise for the chronically dysfunctional cardiopulmonary patient have been relatively well documented, such principles for the acutely dysfunctional cardiopulmonary patient are blatantly lacking in the literature. Exercising the acute patient is a complex matter requiring an integration of exercise principles with the primary disease pathophysiology and the pathophysiology of deconditioning. Despite the paucity of information, a rational basis for exercise prescription for these patients can be extrapolated from the physiologic literature and the underlying pathophysiologic mechanisms of cardiopulmonary dysfunction.

Optimizing oxygen transport is the primary goal of exercise prescription[3,4] in the short and long term for patients with acute or chronic cardiopulmonary dysfunction. These patients can be viewed as being at opposite ends of the same continuum. The factors limiting or enhancing O_2 transport, however, are clearly different in these two groups. In the acute patient, deconditioning has been ascribed to orthostatic intolerance and inactivity.[10-12] Both gravitational and exercise stimuli are essential components of the exercise prescription for the acute patient, who typically spends considerable periods of time recumbent. Although chronic patients may be inactive, they typically are not on bed rest. Exercise is primarily limited in these patients by their underlying pathology and secondary deconditioning.[13] Therefore, an exercise stimulus without the need to elicit hemodynamic responses to a gravitational stimulus per se, is the focus of the exercise prescription for chronic stable cardiopulmonary patients.[14,15] These distinctions provide the physiologic bases for exercise prescription in acute and chronic patients.

Because bed rest and inactivity contribute significantly to cardiopulmonary dysfunction regardless of the presence of primary cardiopulmonary pathology, the physiology of bed rest and inactivity need to be addressed in some detail. The negative consequences of bed rest have been recognized for several decades, with a peak in the literature during the 1940s.[16-18] At that time, a large number of war casualities were succumbing to the ill effects of bed rest, whereas soldiers who were ambulated early had a lower incidence of morbidity and mortality.[19] Interest in the effects of bed rest peaked again in the 1960s with the advent of space exploration. A major difficulty in space flight is the effect of prolonged weightlessness on humans, who are designed to be bipedal, upright, and moving in a 1 G gravitational field. Bed rest has been used extensively as a model to research the effects of a weightless or microgravity environment.[8] This body of literature has significiant implications for clinical patient management.[12,20,21]

PHYSIOLOGY OF BED REST, INACTIVITY, AND EXERCISE

Physiologic Effects of Bed Rest

Loss of Gravitational Stimulation

The loss of gravitational stimulation to the cardiovascular system is the primary determinant of bedrest deconditioning and orthostatic intolerance.[10-12,22,23] Orthostatic intolerance is defined as the inability of the cardiovascular system to maintain blood pressure (BP) and adequate cerebral perfusion pressure against gravity.

At rest, the body fluid is maintained in a steady state among the various intra- and extracellular compartments.[8,24-26] Specifically, 70 percent of the total blood volume is contained within the systemic veins, 10 percent within the systemic arteries, 15 percent within the central circulation (the heart and lungs), and 5 percent within the capillaries. The distribution of blood volume is significantly influenced by gravity,[8,27,28] such that when a person assumes the upright position, up to 15 percent (approximately 700 ml) of the blood volume is shifted from the thorax to the legs. Of this 700 ml of venous blood, 60 percent drains from the coronary and pulmonary vasculature. Conversely, when a person assumes the supine position, a significant fluid shift, from the dependent areas into the intrathoracic veins, occurs.

Three mechanisms have been described that counter this hemodynamic fluid shift on standing and maintain normal circulatory status:[6,8,26] (1) an immediate response that occurs within seconds, (2) an intermediate response that occurs within minutes, and (3) a long-term response that occurs over days. In supine position, cardiac output ($\dot{Q}$) and stroke volume (SV) are initially increased due to the significantly increased venous return. To maintain a constant BP, heart rate (HR), diastolic pressure, and peripheral vascular resistance decrease. When a person stands from supine position, fluid shifts to the lower extremities and results in reductions in SV and $\dot{Q}$, which in turn are compensated for by an increase in HR and peripheral vasoconstriction. If the individual continues to stand for 20 minutes, the increased hydrostatic pressure in the legs leads to transudation of the displaced fluid into the dependent interstitial tissues. Within 10 minutes of standing, 10 percent of the plasma volume is shifted; after 20 minutes this volume shift increases to 15 percent. The net effect of this fluid displacement and its transudation into the interstitium is that the absolute volume of the circulation is reduced on prolonged standing and increased on lying down. The long-term mechanism for regulating fluid volume in response to position changes is under neurohumoral control.

Monitoring of well individuals has demonstrated that a negative fluid balance occurs within 24 hours of beginning bed rest.[29] Cardiac filling pressures and SV decrease below normal supine levels. As a result, the individual's ability to compensate for fluid shifts in moving from supine to upright is compromised. An additional concern is that as diuresis occurs, the plasma volume decreases to a greater degree than the red blood cell mass.[30] This in turn increases blood viscosity and the risk of venous stasis and thromboembolism. This problem is further complicated by decreased muscle pump action in the legs during bed rest.

During recumbency, cardiopulmonary work is increased due to the increases in preload and afterload that correspondingly increase the work of breathing (WOB) and the work of the heart. These effects are accentuated in patients with cardiopulmonary involvement, as exemplified by an elevated pulmonary capillary wedge pressure during supine exercise, compared with that in the upright position.[31] Recumbency also increases central venous pressure, which inhibits lymph flow, predisposing the patient to pulmonary edema and further increasing demand on the cardiopulmonary system due to a diffusion defect and increased WOB.[32,33] This increase in cardiopulmonary demand may contribute to the fatigue experienced by hospitalized patients. Concomitantly, the increased HR associated with orthostatic intolerance has been reported to be the basis of postoperative fatigue.[22] These adverse effects of recumbency on cardiopulmonary function were recognized in the 1950s in studies of cardiac patients, unequivocally supporting the importance of early ambulation. The use of "chair" treatment was advocated as a means of reducing the work of the heart and WOB.[23] Thus, postoperative fatigue, the incidence of cardiopulmonary complications, and the sequelae of elevated central venous pressure are effectively minimized by promoting the upright position in the hospitalized patient.

Numerous bedrest studies have examined the relationship between orthostatic tolerance and exercise tolerance. These studies have been reviewed by Blomqvist, Convertino, and Sandler.[7,8,29] Some studies report a positive relationship between the two variables and attribute this to the increased circulating blood volume associated with physical conditioning. Other studies, however, report an inverse relationship or no relationship. These conflicting results have three significant clinical implications. First, exercise tolerance per se is not a valid predictor of orthostatic tolerance. Second, specific measures to counter orthostatic intolerance must involve a gravitational stimulus to evoke fluid shifts from the central to peripheral circulation during periods of bed rest. And third, exercise alone does not elicit the appropriate stimulus for countering orthostatic intolerance. Exercise in the supine position during bed rest does *not* prevent orthostatic intolerance, whereas intermittent daily sitting or standing is effective.[27,34]

Because of the significant hemodynamic consequences of orthostatic intolerance, several investigators[10–12,22,23,35] concluded that impairment of blood pressure– and volume-regulating mechanisms in response to position-induced fluid shifts has a *more* significant role in deconditioning during bed rest than physical inactivity. The direct relationship of microgravity to bedrest deconditioning provides strong evidence that measures to counter the effects of microgravity, (i.e., sitting and early ambulation) are an essential step toward enhancing O_2 transport and preventing cardiopulmonary complications in all hospitalized patients.

Loss of Exercise Stimulation

Next to the loss of gravitational stimulation, the loss of exercise stimulation is a principal determinant of bed rest deconditioning. Since the 1950s, innumerable studies have examined the physiologic effects of inactivity during bed rest. Because this work has been reviewed extensively elsewhere,[19,36–39] the effects of inactivity are only briefly discussed below.

Physiologic Effects of Inactivity

Negative effects of inactivity during bed rest include (1) increased resting and submaximal HR[40]; (2) decreased maximum oxygen uptake ($\dot{V}O_2$ max)[41]; (3) reduced total blood volume, plasma volume, and hematocrit[40–42]; and (4) increased blood viscosity and decreased venous blood flow, hence increased risk of thromboembolism.[34,43] The most profound effects on the pulmonary system include a reduction in functional residual capacity (FRC), residual volume (RV), and forced expiratory volumes (FEV).[44–48] A reduction in FRC predisposes the individual to airway closure, ventilation and perfusion ($\dot{V}_A:\dot{Q}$) inequality, and thus impaired O_2 transport.[49–51] The decrease in FRC in supine position compared within sitting position has been attributed to both decrease in thoracic volume and an increase in thoracic blood volume, hence pulmonary venous engorgement.[50] Thus, alveolar–arterial oxygen (A–aO_2) difference and arterial oxygen tension (PaO_2) are reduced during periods of bed rest.[52–54] With respect to the musculoskeletal system, muscle mass and strength are reduced and bone demineralization ensues.[40,55,56] Joint contractures, skin lesions, and decubitus ulcers may also occur during periods of inactivity.[57] Central nervous system changes include slowed electrical activity of the brain, emotional and behavioral changes, slowed reaction times, sleep disturbance, and impaired psychomotor performance.[57–59] Metabolic changes that occur during periods of inactivity include increased calcium excretion from bone loss and increased nitrogen excretion secondary to protein loss from atrophying muscle.[40,55,60] Additionally, bed rest has been associated with a reduction in antibody defense mechanisms, hence an increased risk of infection.[61] Of clinical significance is the fact that cardiopulmonary and cardiovascular deterioration occur at a faster rate than musculoskeletal and psychological deterioration, and that the rate of recovery from the ill effects of bed rest is generally slower than the rate of impairment.[62,63] Many of these findings on the effects of bed rest are from studies performed on healthy young people. These effects have been reported to be magnified in elderly persons.[64]

Physiologic Effects of Exercise

Patients with Cardiopulmonary Dysfunction

To evaluate the acute and long-term exercise responses of patients with cardiopulmonary dysfunction, normal exercise responses are considered in light of each patient's cardiopulmonary pathology as discussed in Chapters 2 and 3.

In patients with cardiopulmonary dysfunction, the etiology of each patient's dysfunction primarily determines the acute and long-term exercise responses that can be expected. Other factors, however, also contribute. To establish what factors are operative, the following questions have to be answered:

1. Is the cardiopulmonary dysfunction acute, chronic, or both, and what are the underlying primary pathophysiologic mechanisms involved?
2. To what degree is this dysfunction further exacerbated by recumbency and inactivity?

3.   Is this dysfunction even further exacerbated by extrinsic and intrinsic factors?

Both extrinsic and intrinsic factors are detailed in Table 8-1. Identification of the specific underlying pathophysiologic mechanisms at each of these levels that contribute to cardiopulmonary dysfunction is essential for efficacious exercise prescription.

For a detailed account of the multitude of cardiopulmonary pathologies and resultant responses to exercise, see Chapter 3 and several reviews on this subject.[65–68] This body of literature shows that the exercise responses, acute and long term, differ significantly depending on the underlying pathology. For example, patients with chronic airflow limitation show increases in exercise duration and subjectively report reduced distress following training.[14,69] The mechanisms for this improvement, however, are different from those observed in healthy persons in that airflow-limited patients are frequently unable to achieve training thresholds of sufficient intensity to elicit normal training responses such as increased $\dot{V}O_2$ max and anaerobic threshold.[70] Interestingly,

Table 8-1. Factors Contributing to
Cardiopulmonary Dysfunction

Primary cardiopulmonary pathophysiology
    Acute
    Chronic
    Acute and chronic
Cardiopulmonary dysfunction secondary to
    Bed rest
    Inactivity
Cardiopulmonary dysfunction secondary to
    extrinsic factors
    Effects of surgery
    Incisions
    Invasive lines
    Monitoring equipment
    Medications
    Intubation
    Mechanical ventilation
    Suctioning
    Pain
    Anxiety
    Reduced arousal
    Multisystem complications
    Fixation devices, casts, splints
Cardiopulmonary dysfunction secondary to
    intrinsic factors
    Age
    Smoking history
    Obesity
    Nutritional status
    Musculoskeletal deformity
    Fluid and electrolyte balance
    Previous medical and surgical history
    Natural immunity

however, some studies have shown reduced HR, systolic blood pressure (SBP), and rate pressure product (RPP) at submaximal exercise loads.[71,72] (RPP = [HR $\times$ SBP] $\div$ 100, which yields an index of $\dot{Q}$ and myocardial oxygen consumption.) Explanations for improvement in exercise tolerance include improved aerobic capacity, which could occur in mild disease. In moderate to severe disease more likely explanations include desensitization to dyspnea, increased motivation, improved movement efficiency, and improved ventilatory muscle indurance.[73-76]

The acute exercise responses of patients with interstitial lung disease (ILD), reviewed by Chung and Dean,[66] include rapid, shallow breathing; reduced cardiac output ($\dot{Q}$); and increased pulmonary vascular resistance, pulmonary artery pressure, and right ventricular work.[77-79] The training responses of ILD patients have not been compared with the training responses of patients with chronic airflow limitation; thus, principles for prescribing exercise for ILD patients are lacking.[66]

The ventilatory muscles primarily serve an endurance function, which may be compromised by primary lung disease. Both ventilatory muscle endurance and strength have been reported to increase in healthy persons following a running program.[80] Keens et al.[81] reported that patients with cystic fibrosis exhibited greater ventilatory muscle endurance than healthy subjects (a discrepancy probably explained by the chronic stress of breathing against an inspiratory resistive load) and that ventilatory muscle endurance was further increased in response to upper extremity aerobic training. Pardy and Leith[82] reviewed the effects of ventilatory muscle training versus the physiologic adaptations of the ventilatory muscles to whole-body training. Although these investigators concluded that ventilatory muscle training may have a role in improving ventilatory muscle performance at rest and during exercise in some patients with chronic airflow limitation, they argued that the role of ventilatory muscle training is unclear for other cardiopulmonary conditions, that the indications for training have not been elucidated, and that some patients may require rest rather than exercise to enhance the performance of their ventilatory muscles (see Ch.7).

Of additional clinical importance is the effect of exercise on mucociliary transport. A study of healthy young adults by Wolff et al.[83] provided conclusive evidence that exercise, as compared with eucapnic hyperventilation, significantly increased secretion clearance from all lung zones. In addition, exercise is increasingly considered to be the most effective means of secretion mobilization and clearance in cystic fibrosis patients.[84-86] Possible explanations for the beneficial effects of exercise on reducing secretion accumulation and stimulating coughing include (1) increases in respiratory volumes, breathing frequency, and flow rates[87] and (2) exercise-induced bronchodilation.[88] Exercise hyperpnea also enhances the distribution of ventilation ($\dot{V}e$) by the recruitment of alveoli and by increasing the area of $\dot{V}_A:\dot{Q}$ matching in the lung.[89] Conversely, voluntary hyperpnea (i.e., breathing exercises) may overexpand already open alveoli, thus contributing less to the enhancement of the distribution of $\dot{V}_A:\dot{Q}$ matching and hence, gas exchange.[90] Thus, consistent with the literature, Orenstein et al.[91] have advocated that response to exercise, rather than sputum volume and pulmonary function tests, can provide a better index of the functional status of cystic fibrosis patients.

Patients with cardiac involvement such as coronary artery disease are capable of increasing symptom-limited $\dot{V}O_2$ and anginal threshold in response to training, and reducing submaximal HR, SBP, and RPP at submaximal work rates.[92] These changes reflect both peripheral adaptations (i.e., enhanced oxygen extraction at the tissue level) and central adaptations (i.e., increased SV as observed in healthy persons). In addition, training may enhance myocardial vascularity and contribute to improved coronary artery collateralization and hence, coronary perfusion.[93,94]

Objective of the Exercise Prescription

Exercise training is a widely accepted means of enhancing O_2 transport in patients with cardiopulmonary disease.[69,95,96] The exercise prescription quantifies the details of the threshold stimulus needed to elicit the physiologic adaptations for optimal O_2 transport. With an understanding of the pathophysiology of cardiopulmonary dysfunction, we can apply the principles of exercise prescription to patients with a wide range of cardiopulmonary dysfunction.

Several factors distinguish the acute patient from either the healthy person or the person with chronic cardiopumonary dysfunction:

1. Management of the acute patient is more complicated by both extrinsic and intrinsic factors (Table 8-1)

2. The contributing factors to acute cardiopulmonary dysfunction are multifactorial, requiring more outcome measures to assess the patient's status and the efficacy of the exercise prescription.

3. Prediction of the exercise response is more complex for the acute patient than for the chronic patient because of the multifactorial nature of the factors contributing to dysfunction.

4. Performing a preliminary exercise test on which to base the exercise prescription may not be feasible.

5. The acute patient's condition changes rapidly. The patient, therefore, is assessed and treated more frequently than the relatively stable chronic patient, requiring the exercise prescription be adjusted frequently to include new or reprioritized means of optimizing O_2 transport. Inadequate O_2 delivery may preclude the use of mobilization in some patients.

These multiple factors must be considered on an individual basis when prescribing exercise for the acute patient.

Conditioning and exercise performance are primarily enhanced by a threshold exercise stimulus that the individual is exposed to over a prescribed period of time.[97] Furthermore, in the acute patient, conditioning also includes exposure to gravitational stimulus.[10,11,21–23] The question then arises as to what physiologic reserves the patient can muster to effect physiologic adaptation to exercise stimulation. Further, what constitutes an optimal stimulus for enhancing performance for a given patient? What are the clinical decision making criteria used in making the exercise prescription? These questions are addressed in the following sections for both the acute and chronic patient. How the exercise prescription is applied and progressed for each type of patient is also discussed.

EXERCISE PRESCRIPTION IN ACUTE CONDITIONS

Defining the Indications

The indications for mobilization of the patient with acute cardiopulmonary dysfunction reflect the larger number of underlying mechanisms contributing to cardiopulmonary dysfunction and O_2 transport. Mobilization may enhance O_2 transport secondary to its direct effects on:

1. $\dot{V}e$ and its distribution
2. gas exchange
3. perfusion of the lungs
4. tissue perfusion[44,98,99]
5. orthostatic tolerance[11,34,43]
6. movement efficiency[100]
7. lymphatic drainage[32]
8. secretion mobilization and removal[83–85,87,90]
9. countering the effects of anesthesia and surgery[46,101–106]
10. enhancing chest tube drainage
11. reducing the risks of bed rest and inactivity.[9,16–18,32,107]

The various mechanisms that contribute to a patient's cardiopulmonary dysfunction determine the appropriate measures employed to specifically assess the efficacy of exercise.[108] Critically ill patients are supported by intensive monitoring, which provides the information for a detailed baseline assessment and evaluation of response to treatment.[109,110] For example, vital signs, electrocardiograms (ECG), fluid intake and output, fluid and electrolyte balance, blood work, blood gases, radiographs, and hemodynamic monitoring are frequently assessed. The monitoring capabilities of the intensive care unit, and the objective test results, and daily monitoring recorded in the chart can be exploited for patient evaluation and guiding modifications in the exercise prescription.

Defining the Parameters

Because there are no specifically defined upper and lower limits of the acute patient's exercise response to serve as the basis for the exercise prescription, determining safe, effective treatment is challenging. Such predefined limits provide the basis for exercise prescription in chronically ill and healthy persons.[111] In the acute setting, a decision is made each time the patient is seen to determine the optimal therapeutic stimulus[112] required to enhance O_2 transport and provide an appropriate gravitational stimulus. The patient's optimal response most often falls within a narrow range between under- and over-treatment.

Determination of the therapeutic range of response to gravity and exercise stimuli for the acute patient is based on a prediction of the patient's response rather than on an exercise prescription derived from a symptom-limited test. The accuracy of this prediction depends on consideration of several factors, including the evaluator's understanding of exercise physiology/pathophysiology, the patient's physiologic state related to his pathology and response to bedrest, the extrinsic and intrinsic factors related to the patient's current and past medical/surgical conditions, and the patient's personal characteristics (see Table 8-1). Given these factors, the therapeutic measures (i.e., exercise prescription) are selected in an effort to correct, minimize, or prevent the detrimental effects of pathology and bedrest without unduly stressing any system beyond its safety limits.

For healthy persons, components of the exercise prescription are based on the actual maximum HR, BP, respiratory rate (RR), ECG, oxygen saturation (SaO_2) and symptomatic response to exercise, and include the type of exercise, its intensity, duration, frequency, course, and the plan for progression.[111,113] According to the guidelines of the American College of Sports Medicine,[114] to achieve cardiopulmonary conditioning, the individual trains at a heart rate that is 70 to 85 percent of the maximal HR achieved in the pretraining exercise test at peak work rate. Working at 70 to 85 percent of this HR range in healthy persons is equivalent to working at 60 to 70 percent of their $\dot{V}O_2$ max. The recommended duration and frequency of exercise is 30 to 40 minutes per session 3 to 5 times per week. Based on this prescription, aerobic training effects can be observed in 6 to 8 weeks.[111]

These parameters and recommendations assume (1) the goal of exercise is aerobic conditioning, (2) the individual is able to perform aerobic exercise at 60 to 70 percent of $\dot{V}O_2$ max, and (3) the major stimulus increasing O_2 demand is the volitional exercise being performed. Most often none of these presumptions is accurate in the acutely ill patient. Pathology commonly increases O_2 demand at rest; impairs efficiency of activity, increasing the O_2 demand for a given activity; and lowers the $\dot{V}O_2$ max of the individual. Therefore, mobilization for the acute patient mandates accurate assessment of (1) each system's current level of impairment, (2) its capacity to respond to stress, and (3) the factors that will enhance or prevent that response.

Considering the multiplicity of mechanisms that may contribute to the patient's underlying pathophysiology, what type of exercise stimulus will safely and optimally enhance the acutely ill patient's O_2 transport? Possible considerations include

1. positioning to improve $\dot{V}_A:\dot{Q}$ matching, and reduce work of breathing, etc.
2. active positioning to stimulate $\dot{V}e$, deep breathing, secretion mobilization and coughing, and cardiac output

3. sitting up and dangling the legs or transferring to a chair to invoke gravitational and cardiopulmonary responses

4. standing and walking to achieve increased O_2 consumption and transport and for musculoskeletal/gravitational benefit

5. some combination of these

What are the appropriate measures to evaluate treatment response and outcome, immediate posttreatment effects, and the long-term effects between treatments? Simple clinical measures of HR and heart rhythm, RR, pattern and use of ventilatory muscles, BP, SaO_2, and symptoms are most useful. The optimal frequency and intensity of mobilization and the optimal length of the treatment are based on each patient's clinical responses.

For acute patients, mobilization focuses on functional activities that will elicit gravity and exercise responses, specifically, the response to the gravity stimulus conditions by the patient to accommodate to position changes. Optimizing orthostatic tolerance in turn optimizes the acute patient's exercise responses. The exercise stimulus and intensity are selected to increase $\dot{V}e$ and $\dot{Q}$ such that exercise responses are within the predetermined safe therapeutic range. This raises additional questions regarding the intensity of the gravity and exercise stimuli (e.g., what constitutes the therapeutic range?). What constitutes the subtherapeutic zone and the supratherapeutic or danger zone? General guidelines for appropriate and inappropriate responses are presented in Chapters 2 and 3. At the low end of the mobilization continuum, turning in bed with assistance may constitute adequate gravity and exercise stimuli for one patient; however, these stimuli elicit subtherapeutic responses for another patient who is self-positioning with ease. It is crucial, therefore, that gravity and exercise stimuli are prescribed individually for each patient to generate a safe and optimal therapeutic response.

Criteria that may be appropriate for chronic patients are not as applicable to the acute patient in that the cardiopulmonary and cardiovascular responses may be generally more abnormal and more labile in acute patients. A decision is then made regarding the patient's capacity for oxygen delivery to the tissues and whether an increase in metabolic demand elicited by an exercise stimulus, no matter how minimal, can be tolerated and sustained. This is essential if the prescription of exercise to effect acute cardiopulmonary responses, is to be optimal, that is, maximal benefit-to-risk ratio. The acute exercise response is compared to the patient's pre-exercise status. The exercise stimulus is then set at a threshold that elicits a physiologic demand for a given patient but is below the threshold of the signs and symptoms listed below:

HR: sinus rhythm, rate less than 85 percent of maximum predicted
RR: 16 to 30 breaths per minute
Respiratory pattern: coordinated without use; accessory; symmetrical
BP: rising with increasing workload, less than 200/100
SaO₂: greater than 85 percent on room air
Symptoms: less than moderate dyspnea; no angina, dizziness, nausea, cyanosis, severe pain, or discomfort

Patients who are able to ambulate in the hallway with minimal assistance receive prescriptions focusing on the speed and duration of the walk, with monitoring to assure that vital signs, ECG, and SaO_2 remain within acceptable limits yet effect increases in $\dot{V}e$ and $\dot{Q}$. The classic unstructured low-intensity hallway ambulation is not considered a potential therapeutic intervention and does not constitute an effective use of the therapist's expertise and time.[112] The goals of exercise prescription for hallway ambulation are primarily to provide sufficient intensity and duration to prevent deconditioning and, when possible, to increase endurance. Conversely, without appropriate monitoring, excessive cardiopulmonary work in hospitalized acute patients may be elicited by what appears to be an innocuous exercise stimulus.[115] Excessive energy expenditure and undue fatigue can result, for example, from biomechanical inefficiency during ambulation[100] (surgical patients are encouraged to relax the upper body and to avoid clutching pillows or equipment). In part, this can be visually assessed by the patient's facial expression, the quality of gait, and upper limb and trunk rigidity.[116] The therapeutic response will be enhanced if exercise is synchronized with the peak effectiveness of pain medications, the patient is reassured and not anxious, and the patient is fully aroused and aware of what is taking place.

Clinical Considerations

Mode

An important consideration in mobilizing patients is whether the patient is a candidate for frequent position turns in bed, versus sitting up and dangling the legs over the bed, sitting at bedside and walking, or walking and climbing stairs. Positioning and mobilization of the patient are inseparable principles of cardiopulmonary treatment, as each has a unique contribution in optimizing O_2 transport (see Ch. 5). A guiding principle in selecting the appropriate activity is to determine whether the patient can walk, barring absolute contraindications, without being distressed or exhibiting an untoward exercise response (disproportionate HR increase, fall in SBP, plummeting PaO_2, etc.), walking being considered an act of relatively high energy demand for the acute patient. If ambulation is performed very slowly with frequent rests and still generates unsafe responses, then an activity with a relatively lower energy demand, yet still sufficient to elicit a therapeutic response, is selected (e.g., sitting at bedside with some very short assisted walks). If a patient tolerates low-level ambulation with minimal, appropriate physiologic response, then prolonging the duration of the walks or adding stair climbing, for example, may be indicated to provide a higher exercise intensity, provided vital signs and subjective responses remain within therapeutic limits. Altering the rate of walking or stair climbing can be effectively used as a means of adjusting the work load to meet the prescribed intensity. Regardless of the activity, slumped sitting or standing postures may compromise lung volumes[117] and are to be avoided.

Patients in the intensive care unit and others who are severely ill are prime candidates for succumbing to the ill effects of bed rest and inactivity, and these effects are likely to be aggravated when superimposed on primary cardiopulmonary pathology. Regardless of how encumbered by equipment the patient may be, every effort is made to position the patient upright and to approximate standing and ambulation when possible to avoid cardiopulmonary complications.[118,119] The degree of patient participation depends on disease severity. Mechanical ventilation, for example, is not necessarily a contraindication for sitting, standing, and ambulating. Ambulation may facilitate and hasten weaning from mechanical ventilation while minimizing the problems associated with bed and chair rest.[120] Patients with severe ventilatory failure who are nonventilated may benefit from a formalized exercise program. Burns and Jones[120] demonstrated that intermittent ergometer pedalling produced increased PaO_2 and decreased HR, respiratory quotient (RQ), and blood lactate in chronic obstructive pulmonary disease (COPD) patients and severe, prolonged exertional dyspnea. These reports support the contention that severely ill patients can be treated with exercise that is therapeutic and safe. The prophylactic benefits of prescriptive exercise for such patients is immeasurable.

Defining the therapeutic range of objective and subjective responses for the patient is based on several factors as previously described. For the acute patient, subjective measures have an increasingly significant role in addition to objective treatment outcome measures. Subjective measures are discussed in detail in the section on Exercise Prescription for Chronic Conditions.

Intensity and Duration

Both intensity and duration of mobilization are determined by how well the patient tolerated the previous treatment session, any changes in the patient's status since the last session, and the patient's orthostatic and exercise responses to the present session. Two distinguishing features of the exercising acute patient are early fatigue and generally reduced exercise tolerance,[22,57] necessitating shorter treatments with greater frequency. Because acute illness is often associated with rapid changes in the patient's status, frequent assessment is indicated and treatment is constantly modified to address these changes.

The principles of warm-up, cool-down, and recovery that are routinely incorporated into exercise programs for chronic patients are also applicable to the mobilization of the acute patient, given the potential hazards of sudden onset or cessation of exercise for the cardiovascular and cardiopulmonary systems.[121] Exercise sessions include a prolonged warm-up, a short exercise period (if possible, at a prescribed peak load), and a prolonged cool-down. If the patient has an extremely low functional work capacity, the notion of a warm-up and cool-down are still important; however, the delineation of these may be less clear, given the relatively low intensity and short duration of the session. Furthermore, in the severe patient, the exercise intensity may be better tolerated if gradually increased in discrete steps, with rest periods between steps.[122]

Frequency

Warm-up, cool-down, and recovery periods permit ongoing assessment of how the patient is tolerating position change and the increasing metabolic demand of an exercise stimulus. Periodic rests within a treatment session provide an additional clue as to whether the patient recovers predictably from an increased physiologic load. Also, prescribed intermittent rest enables the patient with low functional capacity to prepare for the next exercise load, and for the physical therapist to establish whether a higher intensity is indicated. A greater energy expenditure over a prolonged period of time may be more beneficial and safer than one long exercise session for the individual with low functional capacity.[123] Untoward exercise responses may occur during recovery from an exercise stimulus; thus, a recovery period with monitoring will help establish how well the patient tolerated the session and whether the parameters of the current treatment session are appropriate. This determination in part provides the basis of the exercise parameters for the next treatment.

Applying the Prescription

Application of the exercise prescription consists of appropriate monitoring of the patient when mobilization is instituted to ensure the optimal therapeutic intensity, and determining the indications for, and the methods of exercise prescription progression.

The most readily available pre- and posttreatment outcome measures that offer considerable information about the patient's physiologic capacity to respond therapeutically and safely to a given mobilization stimulus include HR, SBP, mean arterial pressure (MAP), RPP, SaO_2, breathing pattern, and RR. Resting measures are taken after a prolonged period (e.g., 3 minutes of quiet sitting or lying).[124,125] Even when mobilizing the acute patient, calculation of the age-predicted maximum heart rate (APMHR) can be informative in estimating the intensity of the mobilization stimulus (220 − 2/3 [age]).[97,111] During exercise, the HR is taken and its proportion of APMHR is calculated. Thus, the intensity of dangling the legs, walking, or climbing stairs can be gauged in part by whether the HR is within an optimal therapeutic range (i.e., the intensity is sufficient to elicit an exercise response, this demand can be met and tolerated physiologically by the patient, and it incurs minimal risk). Similarly BP, SaO_2, RR, and ventilatory pattern can be monitored to assess if the exercise intensity produces physiologic changes indicating intolerance of the exercise stimulus (see Ch. 3). The specific therapeutic ranges for various cardiopulmonary and cardiovascular parameters need to be established individually for each patient.

Inspection of the patient, particularly facial expression, color, verbalization, degree of alertness, posture, and freedom of movement are additional indexes of exercise tolerance and the appropriateness of the exercise intensity. These subjective parameters yield information about what factors require modification to contribute to a more effective and tolerable treatment response that would be more beneficial to the patient. Such factors include adequacy of pain control, reduction of anxiety about potential negative effects of movement on surgical incisions, and amelioration of a general unrelaxed or agitated state. The patient's exercise responses, including the warm-up and cool-down periods, are continuously compared with that predicted for the individual for the prescribed exercise parameters. That is, are the exercise responses appropriate considering the patient's current status; the time of day; other procedures the patient may have had; medications; and the patient's general level of comfort, pain, anxiety; and so forth? Are the exercise responses consistent with those predicted? If not, why not? What are the implications for progression of the prescription?

Because of the dynamic and at times unpredictable course of acute illness (i.e., progressive improvement, exacerbations and remissions, progressive deterioration, or a patient whose condition remains stable regardless of where that patient is on the recovery curve), the indications for the progression of the exercise prescription and redefining its parameters depend on the outcome of frequent assessments of treatment outcome. These decisions are based on the answers to the following questions:

1. Which components of oxygen transport were, continue to be, or are now impaired and what are the pathophysiologic mechanisms of the cardiopulmonary impairments (e.g., a ventilatory pump impairment produced by fatigued ventilatory muscles or impaired gas exchange due to consolidated alveolar spaces)?

2. What components of the exercise prescription will best address each of the underlying pathophysiologic mechanisms contributing to impaired O_2 transport (e.g., work/rest interval training for the ventilatory muscles or positioning for improved $\dot{V}_A:\dot{Q}$ matching?

3. Which aspects of mobilization have been previously effective with this patient and why were these effective? In the critically ill patient, the intermittent work/rest mobilization regimen may be progressed by increasing the duration of the work, reducing the rest periods, and increasing the overall duration of the session.[122]

4. Which aspects of mobilization were less effective and why? The noncritical acute patient may be able to tolerate an exercise intensity that produces a HR response at the low end of the HR range and an exercise duration ranging from several to 30 minutes. The exercise prescription must increase the intensity and the duration for further improvements.

5. What other explanations are there (e.g., medical surgical, or social) for the patient's treatment response or lack of it?

6. Overall, what implications do these factors have for progression of the exercise prescription and changing the parameters of this prescription?

Thus, on the basis of ongoing patient evaluation, treatment response and analysis of the underlying pathophysiology of impaired O_2 transport, mobilization can be directed toward the underlying problems and prescribed specifically for each acute patient.

EXERCISE PRESCRIPTION FOR CHRONIC CONDITIONS

Defining the Indications

The primary objective of exercise prescription for patients with chronic cardiopulmonary dysfunction is comparable to that for the acute patient, specifically to enhance exercise performance, hence function, by enhancing O_2 transport. The exercise responses of the chronic patient, however, are distinct from those of the acute patient or the healthy person. Further, the type and degree of physiologic adaptation that will occur with an exercise program depends on the individual's underlying pathophysiology and physiologic reserves.

Dyspnea and reduced endurance are the primary complaints of patients with chronic cardiopulmonary dysfunction.[13,14,126-129] Frequently these complaints are associated with abnormalities in pulmonary function and gas exchange at rest and particularly during exercise.[130] The etiology of dyspnea includes such mechanisms as abnormal control of breathing, inappropriate sense of respiratory load, excessive $\dot{V}e$ in relation to maximum breathing capacity, abnormal length–tension relationships of the respiratory muscles, abnormal chest wall mechanics, and respiratory muscle fatigue.[3,13,126] Establishing the pathophysiologic mechanisms underlying the cardiopulmonary dysfunction and those links in the O_2 transport chain that are defective provides the basis for predicting the patient's responses to both acute exercise and training.

The parameters of the exercise prescription for the patient with chronic cardiopulmonary dysfunction are determined from a clinical exercise test.[4,67] The purpose of the exercise test is to determine how a patient's exercise responses differ from normal and to diagnose the specific limitations to exercise. Further, defects in O_2 transport may become apparent only when the patient is exposed to increased metabolic demand during exercise.[130,131] This information provides the basis for the prescription of an exercise program and, in addition, identifies what physiologic adaptations to exercise can be expected. Thus, the type of exercise test conducted depends on the information that is required to prescribe an optimally therapeutic and safe program for a given patient. Regardless of the type of test selected, however, standardization of the procedures and scrupulous attention to the quality of the measures are essential to maximize the reliability and validity of the exercise test.[67] The selection and specifications of the exercise test are based on the history, laboratory investigations including x-rays and scans, and the assessment.

Exercise Testing

Mode and Methodologic Considerations

Exercise testing and training are associated with some risk. To minimize this risk, guidelines have been established to determine whether an exercise test is indicated,[130] and to determine when exercise should be discontinued by the tester.[67] Absolute contraindications to testing imply that the patient should definitely not be tested, whereas relative contraindications imply that the patient may be tested if the relative contraindication is controlled, and if the appropriate personnel are present for monitoring the patient and making decisions during the test. Other than upon abnormal exercise responses, exercise tests are typically terminated at the patient's symptom-limited maximum oxygen uptake ($SL\dot{V}O_2$ max) (i.e., in response to exhaustion, fatigue, exertional dyspnea, or at some arbitrary submaximal level, such as at 85 percent of APMHR).[15,70] A sign-limited test is one terminated because the patient exceeded the limits of vital signs or cardiac arrhythmias occurred. Neither the sign nor symptom-limited test constitutes a $\dot{V}O_2$ max test. The endpoint of a true physiologic $\dot{V}O_2$ max test is one in which a further increase in work rate does not result in further increase in $\dot{V}O_2$.[132] Considering it as such will lead to erroneous interpretation of the test results and erroneous predictions about the effect of training based on a proportion of the peak load achieved in the exercise test.

The exercise test can be conducted with varying degrees of sophistication, ranging from a 12-minute walk test[133] or some modification, to oxygen consumption studies with blood gas analysis and cardiac catheterization.[67] Other variants include the symptom-limited exercise test versus the steady-state exercise test, and the intermittent versus continuous exercise test. The advantages and disadvantages of these different levels and variants of exercise testing are discussed below.

Walk Tests.   Although tests such as the 12-minute walk test[133] and its modifications (3- or 6-minute walk tests) have several advantages, particularly for patients with poor exercise tolerance, and are straightforward to perform, they are prone to methodologic problems. Their advantages include the fact that they can be carried out in a wide variety of settings, can be performed by one tester, are an activity familiar to the patient, and are easily measured before, during, and after the test. The patient is asked to walk as far as possible in 12 minutes (or 3 or 6 minutes) such that by the end of the test the patient could not have covered more ground in that time. The patient can slow down or stop during the test as necessary. Because the intensity of this test is not controlled (i.e., there is no warm-up, graded increase in exercises intensity, or cool-down), the test is potentially hazardous. Thus, adequate screening of patients beforehand is needed to ensure that a test not conforming to exercise testing standards with respect to optimizing performance and safety is in fact indicated. Patients should be closely monitored, given that this test can elicit near maximal exercise responses in some patients.

Another methodologic difference in conducting the walk test is the number of times it should be repeated to enhance the validity of the test results. On the basis of their repeated measures data, McGavin et al.[133] advocated repeating the 12-minute walk test on two different days and using the result from the second day because of an apparent learning effect. Other studies, however, do not adhere to this recommendation. For example, Cockcroft et al.[134] repeated the test on the same day and averaged the distance covered. Repeating the test without at least 24 hours between tests is a violation of the testing procedures described by McGavin et al.[133] In addition to jeopardizing the validity of the test results, repeating the test on the same day may be an unsafe practice particularly in an older, deconditioned patient population. Clinicians should consider methodologic and validity issues related to conducting versions of the 12-minute walk test in patients with cardiopulmonary dysfunction, or the results of the test may not be reproducible or valid. Reliability and validity considerations have significance in the interpretation of the exercise test results as demonstrated by Cockcroft et al.,[134] who found that other treatment outcome measures, such as treadmill exercise performance and resting lung function, were unchanged with training, based on pre- and posttraining test values. The investigators had based their conclusions regarding the value of the exercise regimen for chronic patients solely on the results of the 12-minute walk test.

Treadmill and Cycle Ergometer Tests.   Objective standardized tests can be achieved using a treadmill or cycle ergometer. These instruments should be calibrated on a regular basis to standardize work rates and minimize the degree of systematic error.[67] The effect of practice and habituation on arousal and exercise test performance has been documented.[135] One or more practice sessions should be carried out prior to the day of the exercise test. If the treadmill is used and the patient needs hand rail support, only finger support should be used.[136] If the cycle ergometer is selected, the seat is adjusted so the legs are almost fully extended when the pedals are in the lowermost position, and the handle bars are adjusted to waist height for optimal cycling efficiency.[67] Toe clips or foot straps are used to promote uniform leg work throughout each pedal cycle and for safety reasons. Smoking, eating, and drinking are also controlled for at least 3 hours prior to the exercise test to avoid contamination by these factors of the test results.[125] Miller et al.[108] and Jones[67] have reviewed the issue of quality control in clinical exercise testing. All those involved with exercise testing need to be cognizant of these issues, given that the results of these tests provide a basis for clinical decision making.

Upper extremity ergometry is associated with some unique characteristics. First, upper limb work is associated with a greater cardiovascular demand than lower extremity work,[137–139] increasing the risk of injury or symptomatic limitation for many cardiopulmonary patients, who tend to be older and deconditioned. Second, BP is particularly difficult to measure with increasing work rates because it is more difficult for the patient to maintain cycling cadence while releasing one arm for BP measurement. A possible alternative to measuring brachial pressure is measuring ankle systolic pressure using Doppler ultrasound or photoplethysmography.[140] Ankle systolic pressure, however, is a valid index of systemic pressure only in patients without arterial occlusive disease.[140] Further study about the use of ankle systolic pressure measurements during upper extremity exercise is needed to establish its validity and reproducibility, and to address methodologic issues related to its use in exercise.

Protocols and Measurement

Numerous exercise test protocols have been reported for patients with cardiopulmonary dysfunction.[15,67,108] These tests are usually incremental, starting at a minimal work load and then increasing the load in discrete steps every 2 to 3 minutes until the patient reaches a sign or symptom-limited work rate.

Typically, these increments do not exceed 1 MET (a MET is the amount of oxygen consumed at rest) in patients with compromised exercise tolerance.[67] Conventional monitoring includes both objective measures, such as ECG, SBP, MAP, RPP, RR, breathing pattern, SaO_2, and subjective measures, such as perceived exertion, chest pain, fatigue, leg discomfort, and breathlessness. Measures are recorded every 1 to 2 minutes during the test.

Borg[141,142] originally developed a scale with ratio properties to measure perceived exertion during exercise. Such quasi-objective measures of perceptions of exercise intensity have an important role in exercise testing and in determining exercise intensity.[143] This scale has been modified to measure dyspnea,[144] fatigue,[145] and chest or leg pain[146] during exercise. The patient is encouraged to continue walking or cycling until symptoms develop that prevent further exercise, or until the test is terminated by the tester because the predetermined end-points of the test are reached. Once the termination point is reached, the cool-down commences.

The cool-down period post maximal exercise lasts 10 to 15 minutes, until the ECG and BP stabilize to within 10 percent of baseline values for at least 5 to 10 minutes.[121,147] The patient is monitored in sitting for an additional 10 minutes to ensure that exercise has been tolerated well and that the patient's vital signs and subjective responses have returned to resting levels. The reason the patient cites for terminating the test (e.g., breathlessness, cramp, fatigue, leg pain, chest pain) is recorded.

Test Levels.   Jones[67] has described four levels of exercise testing, beyond the basic clinical exercise test described above, for obtaining a detailed profile of O_2 transport using oxygen consumption studies, blood gas analysis, and arterial catheterization. In addition to the parameters measured in the conventional exercise test, the stage 1 test measures $\dot{V}e$, Vt, RR, $\dot{V}O_2$. Stage 2, 3, and 4 tests are extensions of stage 1. In stage 2 and stage 3, power outputs of one-third and two-thirds the maximum power output achieved in stage 1 are used. These tests are steady-state tests. In stage 2 test, mixed venous PCO_2 and CO are calculated from a rebreath equilibration procedure. The stage 3 and stage 4 tests involve invasive measurements, including blood sampling and arterial catheterization. In the stage 3 test, $PaCO_2$, PaO_2, pH, and plasma lactate are measured. In addition, V_D:Vt (ratio of dead space to tidal volume), P_{AO_2}, and CO, and the venous admixture ratio are obtained. In the stage 4 test, pulmonary vascular pressures are measured directly. The decision as to which of the four tests is indicated is based on the patient's history, assessment, and performance in the stage 1 test. If the mechanism of the patient's exercise-induced cardiopulmonary limitation can be identified from the stage 1 test and if the exercise responses are consistent with those predicted for the patient, no further testing is indicated.

Symptom-Limited Versus Steady-State Tests.   A decision has to be made regarding whether a symptom-limited test or a steady-state test is indicated. The decision depends on the status of the patient and the objectives of the test. A symptom-limited test provides information about the mechanisms of the patient's limitations to exercise. Common complaints cited for terminating a submaximal exercise test include shortness of breath, chest pain, leg pain, muscle cramps, and fatigue. If oxygen consumption studies are included, expired gas analysis provides a detailed profile of a patient's responses to incremental work rates. In addition, such studies can differentiate whether the patient has a pulmonary or cardiac limitation.[108] A steady-state test can be used to assess a patient's ability to maintain a submaximal work rate over an extended period of time. Submaximal exercise testing may be more feasible and practical for older and disabled persons.[125,145,148] Although predictions of maximal work capacity can be determined for some individuals from the results of a submaximal exercise test using a nomogram or extrapolation procedures,[97,108] the purpose of defining maximal work capacity is probably of less value and less valid in patients with chronic cardiopulmonary dysfunction.

Uninterrupted Versus Interrupted Protocols. Clinical exercise testing of patients with chronic cardiopulmonary dysfunction involves the use of either uninterrupted or interrupted protocols. Jones[67] and Frownfelter[147] have advocated uninterrupted exercise testing protocols. Jones recommended the use of an ergometer, as work rates can be more readily quantified and patients do not have to support themselves, and thus, this mode may be safer for severely affected patients.[149] In testing debilitated cardiac patients, others[150–153] have favored the use of a treadmill because walking is a more functional and familiar activity. Frownfelter[147] did not advocate exercise testing for the severely debilitated patient in the traditional sense, although she described assessment and training strategies using target HR parameters recommended for healthy persons (75 to 85 percent of APMHR for such a patient). Because of the increased risk of hypoxemia and cardiac arrhythmias during exercise, some patients may require supplemental oxygen. For the less debilitated patient, Frownfelter[147] recommended a testing protocol starting at 1 mph with 0 percent grade and increasing to a comfortable walking speed, (e.g., 1.5 to 2 mph) to determine at what workload O_2 is required. Grade changes of 2.5 percent are made thereafter and maintained for 3 minutes at each work rate. Barring the patient terminating the test, the test is terminated by the therapist when the patient's SaO_2 drops below 85 percent or he achieves 85 percent of APMHR.

Sheffield and Roitman[122] have advocated the use of interrupted exercise testing protocols. In citing Astrand's findings[123] that interrupted exercise can result in greater energy expenditure than a single prolonged exercise bout, Sheffield and Roitman[122] noted that this principle held for exercise bouts as short as 10 seconds. These investigators stated that by extending the exercise test duration through use of an interrupted testing protocol, valid information on the exercise performance of severely affected patients could be elicited. Mason and Likar[154] reported using 5 minutes of exercise followed by 5 minutes of rest. The exercise intensity was increased for each exercise bout. Hellerstein et al.[155] reported using 6-minute exercise bouts on the ergometer with 4-minute rests between bouts. The test is terminated at an HR of 150 bpm (beats per minute). As with Mason and Likar,[154] the exercise intensity was increased for each exercise bout. Despite its apparent advantages,[123] interrupted exercise testing protocols may pose greater risk to the patient with low functional capacity. The effect of sudden onset and cessation of exercise, particularly at relatively high intensities, for such a patient warrants study.

Exercise testing can be used to derive a dyspnea index (DI).[15,156] The patient walks at a steady state on a treadmill at 2 mph with 0 percent grade.

Expired gas measures are averaged over the portion of the test in which the patient has achieved a steady state. The DI is calculated from the equation

$$DI = (\dot{V}e \div MVV) \times 100\%$$

where MVV (maximum voluntary ventilation) can be calculated from the equation

$$MVV = FEV_1 \times 35$$

Dyspnea is considered severe if the DI exceeds 50 percent, mild to moderate if the DI is between 35 and 50 percent, and is absent if the DI is less than 35 percent. Healthy persons have DIs in the range of 15 to 25 percent.

Terminating the Test

Indications for terminating an exercise test are general signs and symptoms, electrocardiographic signs, HR, and BP.[111,130] General signs and symptoms for stopping exercise include severe dyspnea, dizziness, fainting, onset of cyanosis, sudden onset of pallor and sweating, chest pain suggestive of angina, sudden and disproportionate hyperventilation, and an SaO_2 of less than 85 percent. ECG signs include frequent ventricular premature beats in isolation or runs of three or more; atrial fibrillation; second- or third-degree block; and ischemia-related changes, such as a marked ST segment depression, T wave inversion, or the appearance of a Q wave; and a bundle branch block. Exercise-induced changes in the ST segment of the ECG are frequently associated with myocardial ischemia, and thus are frequently used as an exercise termination criteria. Other factors, however, such as conduction abnormalities, left ventricular hypertrophy, medications, and electrolyte disturbances may also produce ST changes.[157] Thus, these extraneous factors need to be ruled out. BP signs for terminating exercise include a fall in BP below resting level, a fall of more than 20 mmHg after increasing an exercise load, and a systolic pressure greater than 220 mmHg and a diastolic pressure greater than 110 mmHg. The proportion of SBP to peak SBP at 1, 2, and 3 minutes postexercise has been reported to be more sensitive than ECG and angina in detecting coronary artery disease.[158,159] Abnormal proportions are greater than 1.0, 0.9, and 0.8 at 1, 2, and 3 minutes postexercise, respectively. Thus, the relationship of recovery SBP to peak SBP may have some application in monitoring patients with cardiopulmonary dysfunction.

Defining the Exercise Prescription

The components of the exercise prescription include type of exercise, its intensity, duration, frequency, course, and progression. The type of exercise depends on whether the program is supervised or unsupervised, and on the patient's skill level and interest. This section focuses primarily on the patient on a supervised program. The appropriate modifications can be made, however, for the patient on an unsupervised home program. The modifications usually involve (1) a more conservative exercise program than if the program were supervised, (2) self-monitoring strategies, and (3) recording a log.[160]

Mode

Walking and cycling are the two most common activities used in training programs for chronic cardiopumonary patients.[67] However, exercise tests performed on different modalities (e.g., treadmill and ergometer) yield different results,[161] and training on one modality will not necessarily improve performance to the same degree as on another modality.[75,162] Thus, the patient should be exercise tested before and after training on the same modality used for training if a valid index of exercise program effect is to be obtained.

Few studies have examined in detail the role of upper limb testing and training in patients with cardiopulmonary dysfunction. One exception is the work of Keens et al.,[81] which showed improvements in functional work capacity in cystic fibrosis patients following a daily swimming and canoeing program. In addition, O'Hara et al.[163,164] argued that because patients with COPD experience little aerobic training response after endurance training, there may be a role for anaerobic training in these patients. These investigators studied the effect of upper extremity weight training and backpacking on endurance in chronic patients. They observed increases in maximal work capacity and decreases in abnormal lung volumes when these patients trained with weights and backpacks compared with the control condition. One other study by Ries et al.[165] showed that upper extremity training in conjunction with a walking program increased both maximal work capacity and endurance, and decreased fatigue and breathlessness in patients with COPD. No change was observed in expiratory flow rates (FEF) and ventilatory muscle endurance. However, unexpected findings that were not consistent with the existing literature included improved lung capacities and a reduction in chest hyperinflation. These effects were less pronounced in patients who had trained using the walking program alone. The results of these studies confirm the results of previous investigators that upper extremity training may have some role in the long-term training of patients with chronic cardiopulmonary dysfunction.

Intensity

The literature supports that training the patient with chronic airflow limitation is more effective if the intensity of the training program is prescribed on the basis of different criteria than those recommended for healthy persons. Training criteria for healthy persons are based on the presumption that the individual can exercise to an intensity such that HR approximates APMHR. If a patient has particularly mild disease, the criteria used for healthy persons may be used and may produce an aerobic training response, (i.e., 70 to 85 percent of the maximum HR achieved in the symptom-limited exercise test, which is equivalent to 56 to 77 percent of the VO_2 max.[132] Exercising this type of patient continuously in the target HR range of 70 to 85 percent of the symptom-limited heart rate probably elicits an aerobic training response when performed for at least 30 minutes, 3 times a week for 6 to 8 weeks. Patients with significant cardiopulmonary limitations, however, cannot typically reach or maintain this peak level,[14] and so usually cannot tolerate exercising continuously within the parameters for healthy persons. Shephard[166] advocated a target HR of from 50 to 75 percent of the peak HR achieved in the symptom-limited exercise test. This wide range accommodates patients with varying disease severities and functional capacities. It is likely that these patients who are unable to train in the conventional target HR range are not exercising predominantly aerobically, which explains why the literature fails to confirm an aerobic training response in most patients with chronic airflow limitation.

Other training protocols for patients with low functional capacities have emerged from the cardiology literature. For example, Karvonen et al.[167] advocated a target HR range based on resting heart rate plus 60 to 80 percent of the HR reserve, where the HR reserve equals peak HR achieved in the exercise test minus resting heart rate (HR reserve = peak HR − resting HR). Another objective guideline for prescribing exercise intensity is the use of the target MET method.[168] The target MET level for training is defined as:

$$\text{maximum METs} \times (0.6 + [\text{maximum METs} \div 100]).$$

However, this formula assumes a resting O_2 consumption of 3.54 mL/Kg/min and is therefore not useful in the population with moderate or severe cardiopulmonary dysfunction.

In patients with severe disease or whose conditions significantly fluctuate, exercise training intensity is based primarily on subjective ratings. Although attempts have been made to extrapolate objective information from subjective responses to exercise (e.g., 12 to 13, "somewhat hard" on the Borg scale,[141] equivalent to 60 percent of the HR maximum, or 13 to 15 "hard," equivalent to 70 to 85 percent of HR maximum), these guidelines are not likely to be valid for the cardiopulmonary patient who is unable to achieve a true physiologic maximum HR and whose O_2 consumption may be abnormally elevated due to the increased WOB.[169,170] More appropriate for this patient is the use of subjective scales, such as perceived exertion,[143] dyspnea or breathlessness scale,[142,171] fatigue scale,[165] or some combination. The object is to maintain breathlessness, perceived exertion, or fatigue at a constant tolerable level such that power output varies, rather than keeping power output constant.[172] In this way, the patient's WOB is tolerable and the exercise is comfortably endured, thereby maximizing exercise duration.

The work of breathing depends on the rate and depth of breathing, and the resistance to airflow, or the elastic and resistive load of the chest wall and lung. The oxygen cost of WOB at rest is minimal in normals and constitutes 2 percent of the total work during exercise.[132] However, in patients with COPD, WOB is greater at rest due to an increase in mechanical WOB,[129,169,173] and may consume as much as 40 percent of the $\dot{V}O_2$ during exercise. This compares with the 15 percent of $\dot{V}O_2$ consumed by healthy persons. The ability to maintain a high mechanical efficiency of breathing (i.e., high respiratory work output per unit of oxygen required during exercise and at rest) is a significant consideration when attempting to enhance the overall efficiency and work performance of the chronic cardiopulmonary patient.

Duration and Frequency

The duration of the exercise session is initially as short as 1 to 5 minutes if the patient has extremely low endurance, and is increased over time in accordance with the patient's adaptation to the exercise stimulus. A total of 30 to 40 minutes of continuous exercise at the target load is desirable to improve endurance.[15] To achieve this goal, sessions of 1 to 5 minutes' duration are conducted several times daily.[174] Exercise sessions of 30 to 40 minutes are conducted 3 to 5 times a week in keeping with the duration and frequency of training for healthy persons. The shorter the duration of each session, the more frequent the number of sessions needed to elicit physiologic adaptations to training.

Implementing the Prescription

Achieving the benefits of an exercise program depends equally on the development of the prescription and its application. Patients with airway hyperreactivity may benefit from bronchodilator use prior to the exercise and a gradual warm-up, with prolonged exercise of relatively low intensity.[175] Slow warm-up allows for a gradual accommodation of the airways to the demands of exercise, thus reducing adverse symptoms.[176] Exercise-induced bronchospasm occurs more commonly during running and arm-cranking, and less so during swimming and cycling[125]; this will influence modality choice. Exercising in humid, warm environments helps control exercise-induced bronchospasm. The implementation of exercise prescription for any patient should be based on (1) the patient's ability to access the proper environment and modality, (2) the clinical conditions required to enhance performance (medications, oxygen), and (3) the likelihood of goal achievement (intensity, duration, and frequency).

Patients with severe cardiopulmonary dysfunction may benefit from interrupted exercise and an interval training program.[15,123,177,178] A greater net energy expenditure occurs if work is performed in brief spurts separated by rest periods. Pierce et al.[76] observed positive training effects in patients who walked for 2.5 minutes 5 to 10 times daily. Patients rested at least long enough for vital signs to return to baseline. For physiologic adaptations to occur following such low-intensity exercise programs, the patient needs to participate in the program for at least 3 months.[69,70,179]

Pre-exercise Measurements

Pre-exercise measurements are taken to establish a baseline to be used for comparison during exercise. Objective measures to monitor include ECG, BP, MAP, RPP, SaO_2, HR, and breathing pattern. Subjective measures such as perceived exertion, level of breathlessness, and fatigue are also valuable. These parameters are typically recorded every 2 or 3 minutes through all components of the exercise session including recovery.

Warm-up and Cool-down

The warm-up and cool-down periods are critical components of the exercise session. The warm-up typically consists of several minutes of stretching, range of motion exercises, and thoracic mobility exercises, including use of upper extremities, trunk rotation, and calisthenics. The calisthenics are metabolically graded in terms of their energy cost comparable to those described by Weiss and Karpovich.[180] A progressive series of calisthenics prepares the O_2 transport system as a whole for the moderate level of physiologic demand of the exercise prescription. Typically, the warm-up is designed to increase HR, O_2 consumption, and $\dot{V}e$ to some proportion of the peak load in the exercise prescription. Several minutes of cool-down follow the prescribed exercise. The order of the metabolically graded calisthenics performed in the warm-up is reversed in the cool-down to return vital signs to within 10 percent of baseline values and to observe any delayed effects of exercise. Recovery continues until vital signs have returned or stabilized near resting levels for at least 10 minutes. Of the untoward events that are associated with exercise programs, a significant proportion occur during the recovery period. Thus, an adequate recovery period is mandatory.

Prescription Progression

The exercise prescription is progressed in two ways as the patient physiologically adapts to the exercise stimulus: consideration is given to both intensity and duration components. Over the initial course of training, the patient exercises at the lower range of intensity until a total exercise duration of 20 to 40 minutes is achieved as specified by the prescription. Once the duration goal is achieved, the patient progresses toward the middle to upper range of exercise intensity. Finally, once the patient is consistently exercising in the moderate or higher ranges of HR and RR with subjective variables (e.g., breathlessness and fatigue) within tolerable limits, an exercise retest can be performed if necessary to objectively document progress and to change the parameters of the exercise prescription.

Retesting

At the completion of training (when a patient has reached the training goals), a retest is performed to determine the effects of the training program in conjunction with the improvements noted throughout the training period. Physiologic changes that may occur depending on the patient's disease severity include reduced HR, BP, MAP, RPP, and subjective complaints such as dyspnea at submaximal work loads.[70,71] Functional changes are usually reflected by an increase in exercise duration and a decrease in, or increased tolerance of, dyspnea.[134] This improvement, however, may not be manifested by an increase in peak work performance on the incremental symptom-limited posttest for patients with extremely low functional capacities.[134]

Posttest Planning

Appropriate discharge and follow-up plans are made with the patient. The patient is instructed in self-monitoring procedures (e.g., HR and breathlessness), and in maintaining a log of the details (e.g., exercise intensity, duration, and objective and subjective measures) of each training session. Based on the post-test, parameters are established for the home exercise program. The effectiveness of the home program can be evaluated by having the patient return for a retest 3 months after discharge from the supervised exercise program.

SUMMARY

This chapter has described a physiologic framework and the principles for exercise prescription for the patient with impaired O_2 transport. Patients with acute and chronic cardiopulmonary dysfunction should be viewed as being at opposite ends of the same continuum, in that optimal O_2 transport is the prevailing goal in both the short and long term. However, in the acute patient, eliciting both a gravitational and an exercise stimulus is the objective of mobilization. In the chronic patient, eliciting an exercise stimulus is the chief objective. Although principles for exercise conditioning have been documented in the literature for patients with chronic cardiopulmonary dysfunction such as emphysema and chronic bronchitis, these guidelines are less well established for other chronic disorders such as asthma, cystic fibrosis, and restrictive lung disorders. Furthermore, guidelines for mobilizing acute patients are lacking. Thus, this chapter has consolidated the existing physiologic and empirical knowledge on exercise pathophysiology such that principles for exercise prescription can be extrapolated from the chronic patient to the patient with acute cardiopulmonary dysfunction.

Considerable research is needed to refine the principles for exercise prescription for patients with cardiopulmonary dysfunction. With respect to the acute patient, the physiologic principles of mobilization need to be refined in order that exercise can be prescribed more efficaciously; that is, so as to achieve optimal therapeutic effect with the least risk. In large part, this refinement will come from greater understanding of the pathophysiology of cardiopulmonary dysfunction. In addition, extending our knowledge about the exercise responses of patients with chronic cardiopulmonary dysfunction will help refine the indications for testing, and the appropriate training parameters for a given patient.

Given that many critically ill patients can be effectively mobilized and that this should be a treatment priority, research is needed to investigate various adjuncts that may facilitate patients' responses to treatment: pharmacologic agents, the use of kinetic beds, and the use of adaptive aids and devices for assisting mobilization of particularly heavy and difficult patients.

REFERENCES

1. Dantzker DR: The influence of cardiovascular function on gas exchange. Clin Chest Med 4:149, 1983
2. Guy HJB, Prisk GK: Heart–lung interactions in aerospace medicine. p. 519. In Scharf SM, Cassidy SS (eds): Heart–Lung Interactions in Health and Disease. Marcel Dekker, New York, 1989
3. Wasserman KL, Whipp BJ: Exercise physiology in health and disease. Am Rev Resp Dis 112:219, 1975
4. Weber KT, Janicki JS, McElroy PA et al: Concepts and applications of cardiopulmonary exercise testing. Chest 93:843, 1988
5. West JB: Ventilation, Blood Flow and Gas Exchange. 4th Ed. Blackwell Scientific Publications, Oxford, 1985
6. Rowell LB: Human Circulation Regulation During Physical Stress. Oxford University Press Inc., New York, 1986
7. Convertino VA: Aerobic fitness, endurance training, and orthostatic intolerance. Exerc Sport Sci Rev 15:223, 1987
8. Sandler H.: Cardiovascular effects of inactivity. p. 11. In Sandler H, Vernikos J (eds): Inactivity Physiological Effects. Academic Press, Orlando, FL, 1986
9. Saltin B, Rowell LB: Functional adaptations to physical activity and inactivity. Federation Process 39:1,506, 1980
10. Chase GA, Grave C, Rowell LB: Independence of changes in functional and performance capacities attending prolonged bed rest. Aerospace Med 37:1,232, 1966
11. Gaffney FA, Nixon JV, Karlsson ES et al: Cardiovascular deconditioning produced by 20 hours of bedrest with head-down tilt (− 5 degrees) in middle-aged healthy men. Am J Cardiol 56:634, 1985
12. Hahn Winslow E: Cardiovascular consequences of bed rest. Heart Lung 14:236, 1985
13. Loke J, Mahler DA, Man SFP et al: Exercise improvement in chronic obstructive pulmonary disease. Clin Chest Med 5:121, 1984
14. Belman MJ, and Wasserman KL: Exercise training and testing in patients with chronic obstructive pulmonary disease. Basic Resp Dis 10:1, 1981
15. Zadai C: Rehabilitation of the patient with chronic obstructive pulmonary disease. p. 491. In Irwin S, Tecklin JS (eds): Cardiopulmonary Physical Therapy. CV Mosby, St. Louis, 1990
16. Dock W: The evil sequelae of complete bed rest. JAMA 125:1,803, 1944
17. Dripps RD, Waters RM: Nursing care of surgical patients. I. The "Stir-up." Am J Nurs 41:530, 1941

18. Harrison TR: The abuse of rest as a therapeutic measure for patients with cardiovascular disease. JAMA 125:1,075, 1944
19. Browse NL: The Physiology and Pathophysiology of Bed Rest. Charles C Thomas, Springfield, IL, 1965
20. Chobanian AV, Lille, RD, Tercyak A: The metabolic and hemodynamic effects of prolonged bed rest in normal subjects. Circulation 49:551, 1974
21. Ross J, Dean E: Integrating physiological principles into the comprehensive management of cardiopulmonary dysfunction. Phys Ther 69:225, 1989
22. Christensen T, Bendix T, Kehlet H: Fatigue and cardiorespiratory function following abdominal surgery. Br J Surg 69:417, 1982
23. Levine SA, Lown B: "Armchair" treatment of acute coronary thrombosis. JAMA 148:1,365, 1952
24. Berne RM, Levy MN: Cardiovascular Physiology. 4th Ed. CV Mosby, St. Louis, 1981
25. Folkow B, Neil E: Circulation. Oxford University Press, London, 1971
26. Gauer OH, Thron HL: Postural changes in the circulation. p. 2,409. In Hamilton WF (ed): Handbook of Physiology Vol. 3. American Physiological Society, Washington, D.C., 1965
27. Blomqvist CG, Stone HL: Cardiovascular adjustments to gravitational stress. p. 1,025. In Shepherd JT, Abboud FM (eds): Handbook of Physiology. Vol. 2. American Physiological Society, Bethesda, 1983
28. Ziegler MG: Postural hypotension. Annu Rev Med 31:239, 1980
29. Blomqvist CG: Orthostatic hypotension. Hypertension 8:722, 1986
30. Miller PB, Johnson RL, Lamb LE: Effects of four weeks of absolute bed rest on circulatory functions in man. Aerospace Med 35:1,194, 1964
31. Bygdeman S, Wahren J: Influence of body position on the anginal threshold during leg exercise. Eur J Clin Invest 4:201, 1974
32. Allen SJ, Drake RE, Williams JP et al: Recent advances in pulmonary edema. Crit Care Med 15:963, 1987
33. Lai-Fook SJ: Mechanics of the pleural space: fundamental concepts. Lung 165:249, 1987
34. Wenger NK: Early ambulation: the physiologic basis revisited. Adv Cardiol 31:138, 1982
35. Hung J, Goldwater D, Convertino VA et al: Mechanisms for decreased exercise capacity after bed rest in normal middle-aged men. Am J Cardiol 51:344, 1983
36. Birkhead NC, Haupt GJ, Blizzard JJ et al: Effects of supine and sitting exercise on circulatory and metabolic alterations in prolonged bed rest. Physiologist 6:149, 1963
37. Birkhead NC, Haupt GJ, Meyers RN: Effect of prolonged bed rest on cardiodynamics. Am J Med Sci 245:118, 1963
38. Birkhead NC, Haupt GJ, Issekutz B et al: Circulatory and metabolic effects of different types of prolonged inactivity. Am J Med Sci 247:243, 1964
39. Klemic N, Imle PC: Changes with immobility and methods of mobilization. p. 109. In Mackenzie CF (ed): Chest Physiotherapy in the Intensive Care Unit. Williams and Wilkins, Baltimore, 1981
40. Deitrick JE, Whedon GD, Shorr E et al: Effects of immobilization upon various metabolic and physiologic functions of normal men. Am J Med 4:3, 1948
41. Saltin B, Blomqvist G, Mitchell, JH et al: Response to exercise after bed rest and after training. Circulation 38, suppl. VII:S1, 1968
42. Friman G: Effect of clinical bedrest for seven days on physical performance. Acta Med Scand 205:389, 1979

43. Lentz M: Selected aspects of deconditioning secondary to immobilization. Nurs Clin North Am 16:729, 1981
44. Blair E, Hickman JB: The effect of change in body position on lung volume and intrapulmonary gas mixing in normal subjects. J Clin Invest 34:383, 1955
45. Craig DB, Wahba, WM, Dan H: "Closing volume" and its relationship to gas exchange in the seated and supine positions. J Appl Physiol 31:717, 1971
46. Hsu HO, Hickey RF: Effect of posture on functional residual capacity postoperatively. Anesthesiology 44:520, 1976
47. Powers JH: The abuse of rest as a therapeutic measure in surgery. JAMA 125:1,079, 1944
48. Svanberg L: Influence of position on the lung volumes, ventilation and circulation in normals. Scand J Clin Lab Invest 25, suppl.:S7, 1957
49. Risser NL: Preoperative and postoperative care to prevent pulmonary complications. Heart Lung 9:57, 1980
50. Sjöstrand T: Determination of changes in the intrathoracic blood volume in man. Acta Physiol Scand 22:116, 1951
51. Tyler M: The respiratory effects of body position and immobilization. Respir Care 19:472, 1984
52. Cardus D: O_2 alveolar–arterial tension differences after 10 days' recumbency in man. J Appl Physiol 23:934, 1967
53. Clauss RH, Scalabrini BY, Ray JF et al: Effects of changing body positions upon improved ventilation–perfusion relationships. Circulation 37, suppl. 2:S214, 1968
54. Ray JF, Yost L, Moallem S et al: Immobility, hypoxemia, and pulmonary arteriovenous shunting. Arch Surg 109:537, 1974
55. Donaldson CL, Hulley SB, McMillan DE et al: The effect of prolonged simulated non-gravitational environment on mineral balance in the adult male. NASA Contract CR-108314, Moffett Field, CA, 1969
56. Peacock EE: Comparison of collagenous tissue surrounding normal and immobilized joints. Surg Forum 24:440, 1963
57. Rubin M: The physiology of bed rest. Am J Nurs 88:50, 1988
58. Ryback RS, Lewis OF, Lessard CS: Psychobiologic effects of prolonged bed rest (weightless) in young healthy volunteers. Study II. Aerospace Med 42:529, 1971
59. Zubeck JP, MacNeill M: Effects of immobilization: behavioural and EEG changes. Can J Psychol 20:316, 1966
60. Hulley SB, Vogel JM, Donaldson CL et al: The effect of supplemental oral phosphate on the bone mineral changes during prolonged bedrest. J Clin Invest 50:2,506, 1971
61. Ahlinder S, Birke G, Norberg R et al: Metabolism and distribution of IgG in patients confined to prolonged strict bed rest. Acta Med Scand 187:267, 1970
62. Kottke FJ: The effects of limitation of activity upon the human body. JAMA 196:825, 1966
63. Sandler H, Popp RL, Harrison DC: The hemodynamic effects of repeated bed rest exposure. Aerospace Med 59:1,047, 1988
64. Harper CM, Lyles YM: Physiology and complications of bed rest. J Am Geriatr Soc 36:1,047, 1988
65. Bye PTP, Anderson SD, Woolcock AJ et al: Bicycle endurance performance of patients with interstitial lung disease breathing air and oxygen. Am Rev Respir Dis 126:1,005, 1982
66. Chung F, Dean E: Pathophysiology and cardiorespiratory consequences of interstitial lung disease—review and clinical implications. Phys Ther 69:956, 1989

186   *Pulmonary Management in Physical Therapy*

67. Jones NL: Clinical Exercise Testing. 3rd Ed. WB Saunders, Philadelphia, 1988
68. Hanson P (ed): Exercise and the heart. Cardiol Clin 5:147, 1987
69. Lertzman MM, Cherniack RM: Rehabilitation of patients with chronic obstructive lung disease. Am Rev Respir Dis 114:1,145, 1976
70. Brown HV, Wasserman K: Exercise performance in chronic obstructive lung disease. Med Clin North Am 65:525, 1981
71. Bass H, Whitcomb JF, Forman R: Exercise training: therapy for patients with chronic obstructive pulmonary disease. Chest 57:116, 1970
72. Mertens DJ, Shephard RJ, Kavanagh, T: Long-term exercise therapy for chronic obstructive lung disease. Respiration 35:96, 1978
73. Belman MJ, Kendregan BA: Exercise training fails to increase skeletal muscle enzymes in patients with chronic obstructive pulmonary disease. Am Rev Respir Dis 123:256, 1981
74. Belman MJ, Kendregan BA: Physical training fails to improve ventilatory muscle endurance in patients with chronic obstructive pulmonary disease. Chest 81:440, 1982
75. Paez PN, Phillipson EA, Masangkay M et al: The physiologic basis of training patients with emphysema. Am Rev Respir Dis 95:944, 1967
76. Pierce AK, Taylor HF, Miller WF: Responses to exercise training in patients with emphysema. Arch Intern Med 113:78, 1964
77. Jernudd-Wilhelmsson Y, Hornbald Y, Hedenstierna G: Ventilation perfusion relationships in interstitial lung disease. Eur J Respir Dis 68:39, 1986
78. Sturani C, Spyridion P, Galavotti V et al: Pulmonary vascular responsiveness at rest and during exercise in idiopathic pulmonary fibrosis: effects of oxygen and nifedipine. Respiration 50:117, 1986
79. Spiro SG, Dowdeswell IRG, Clark TJH: An analysis of submaximal exercise responses in patients with sarcoidosis and fibrosing alveolitis. Br J Dis Chest 75:169, 1981
80. Robinson EP, Kjeldgäard JM: Improvement in ventilatory muscle function with running. J Appl Physiol 52:1,400, 1982
81. Keens TG, Krastins IRB, Wannamaker FM et al: Ventilatory muscle training in normal subjects and patients with cystic fibrosis. Am Rev Respir Dis 116:853, 1977
82. Pardy RL, Leith DE: Ventilatory muscle training. Respir Care 29:278, 1984
83. Wolff RK, Dolovich MB, Obminski G et al: Effects of exercise and eucapnic hyperventilation on bronchial clearance in man. J Appl Physiol 43:46, 1977
84. Oldenburg FA, Dolovich MB, Montgomery JM et al: Effects of postural drainage, exercise, and cough on mucus clearance in chronic bronchitis. Am Rev Respir Dis 120:739, 1979
85. Stanghelle JK: Physical exercise for patients with cystic fibrosis. Int J Sports Med 9:6, 1988
86. Zach MS, Purrer B, Oberwaldner B: Effect of swimming on forced expiration and sputum clearance in cystic fibrosis. Lancet 2:1,201, 1981
87. Wood RF, Boat TF, Doerschuk CF: State of the art: cystic fibrosis. Am Rev Respir Dis 113:833, 1976
88. Guyton AC: Textbook of Medical Physiology. 5th Ed. WB Saunders, Philadelphia, 1976
89. West JB: Respiratory Physiology: The Essentials. 3rd Ed. Williams and Wilkins, Baltimore, 1985
90. Campbell EJM, Friend J: Action of breathing exercises in pulmonary emphysema. Lancet 1:325, 1955

91. Orenstein DM, Franklin BA, Doerschuk CF et al: Exercise conditioning and cardiopulmonary fitness in cystic fibrosis. Chest 80:392, 1981

92. Laslett L, Paumer L, Amsterdam E: Exercise training in coronary artery disease. In Hanson P (ed): Exercise and the Heart, Cardiol Clin 5:211, 1987

93. Eckstein RW: Effect of exercise and coronary artery narrowing on coronary collateral circulation. Circ Res 5:230, 1957

94. Kramsch DM, Aspen AJ, Abramowitz BM et al: Reduction of coronary atherosclerosis in moderate conditioning exercise in monkeys on an atherogenic diet. N Engl J Med 305:1,483, 1981

95. Hughes RL, Davison R: Limitations of exercise reconditioning in COLD. Chest 83:241, 1983

96. Kattus AA: Exercise Testing and Training of Individuals with Heart Disease or at Risk for Its Development: A Handbook for Physicians. American Heart Association, Dallas, Texas, 1975

97. Åstrand PO, Rodahl K: Textbook of Work Physiology: Physiological Bases of Exercise. 2nd Ed. McGraw-Hill, New York, 1977

98. Alexander IJ, Spencer AA, Parikh RK et al: The role of airway closure in postoperative hypoxaemia. Br J Anaesth 45:34, 1973

99. Sternweiler MRI: Physiotherapy and the South African heart transplantation patient. Phys Ther 48:1,399, 1968

100. Cavanagh PR, Kram R: The efficiency of human movement—a statement of the problem. Med Sci Sports Exerc 17:304, 1985

101. Bassey EJ, Bennet T, Birmingham AT, et al: Effects of surgical operation and bed rest on cardiovascular responses to exercise in hospital patients. Cardiovasc Res 7:588, 1973

102. Bendixen HH, Bullwinkel B, Hedley-Whyte J et al: Atelectasis and shunting during spontaneous ventilation in anaesthetised patients. Anesthesiology 25:297, 1964

103. Chuley M, Brown J, Summer W: Effect of postoperative immobilization after coronary artery bypass surgery. Crit Care Med 10:176, 1982

104. Craig DB: Postoperative recovery of pulmonary function. Anesthes Analg 60:46, 1981

105. Dull JL, Dull WL: Are maximal inspiratory breathing exercises or incentive spirometry better than early mobilization after cardiopulmonary bypass? Phys Ther 63:655, 1983

106. Gyo K: Benign paroxysmal positional vertigo as a complication of postoperative bedrest. Laryngoscope 98:332, 1988

107. Scheidegger D, Bentz L, Piolino G et al: Influence of early mobilization on pulmonary function in surgical patients. Eur J Int Care Med 2:35, 1976

108. Miller WF, Scacci R, Gast JR: Laboratory Evaluation of Pulmonary Function. JB Lippincott, Philadelphia, 1987

109. Norsen LH, Fox GB: Understanding cardiac output and the drugs that affect it. Nursing 15:34, 1985

110. Wiedemann HP, Matthay MA, Matthay RA: Cardiovascular–pulmonary monitoring the intensive care unit. Part 1. Chest 85:537, 1984

111. Blair SN, Painter P, Pate RR et al (eds): Resource Manual for Guidelines for Exercise Testing and Prescription. Lea & Febiger, Philadelphia, 1988

112. Haskell WL: Physical activity and health: need to define the required stimulus. Am J Cardiol 55:4D, 1985

113. Kattus AA: Exercise Testing and Training of Apparently Healthy Individuals: A Handbook for Physicians. American Heart Association, Dallas, Texas, 1972

114. American College of Sports Medicine: Guidelines for Exercise Testing and Prescription. 3rd Ed. Lea & Febiger, Philadelphia, 1986
115. Baruch IM, Mossberg, KA: Heart-rate response of elderly women to nonweight-bearing ambulation with a walker. Phys Ther 63:1,782, 1983
116. Humberstone N: Respiratory assessment. p. 208. In Irwin S, Tecklin JS (eds): Cardiopulmonary Physical Therapy. CV Mosby, St. Louis, 1985
117. Crosbie WJ, Myles S: An investigation into the effect of postural modification on some aspects of normal pulmonary function. Physiotherapy 71:311, 1985
118. Howell S, Hill JD: Acute respiratory care in open heart surgery. Phys Ther 52:253, 1972
119. Ungerman-deMent P, Bemis A, Siebens A: Exercise program for patients after cardiac surgery. Arch Phys Med Rehabil 67:463, 1986
120. Burns JR, Jones FL: Early ambulation of patients requiring ventilatory assistance. Chest 68:608, 1975
121. The exercise training session. p. 355. In Wilson PK, Fardy PS, Froelicher VF (eds): Rehabilitation, Adult Fitness, and Exercise Testing. Lea & Febiger, Philadelphia, 1981
122. Sheffield LT, Roitman D: Stress testing methodology. p. 145. In Sonnenblick EH, Lesch M (eds): Exercise and Heart Disease. Grune & Stratton, Orlando, FL, 1977
123. Åstrand I: Aerobic work capacity in men and women with special reference to age. Acta Physiol Scand, suppl. 169:S1, 1960
124. Angle DP, Baum GL, Chester GH et al: Multidisciplinary treatment of cardiopulmonary insufficiency. 1. Psychosocial aspects of rehabilitation. Psychosom Med 35:41, 1973
125. Shephard RJ, Cox M, Corey P et al: Some factors affecting the accuracy of the Canadian Home Fitness Test scores. Can J Sport Sci 4:205, 1979
126. Burki NK: Dyspnea. Lung 165:269, 1987
127. Killian KJ: Limitation of exercise by dyspnea. Can J Sport Sci 12, suppl. 1:S53, 1987
128. Leblanc P, Bowie DM, Summers E et al: Breathlessness and exercise in patients with cardiorespiratory disease. Am Rev Respir Dis 133:21, 1986
129. Pardy RL, Hussain SNA, Macklem PT: The ventilatory pump in exercise. Clin Chest Med 5:35, 1984
130. Jones NL: Exercise testing. Medicine 22:4,175, 1988
131. Ries AL, Farrow JT, Clausen JL: Pulmonary function tests cannot predict exercise-induced hypoxemia in chronic obstructive pulmonary disease. Chest 93:454, 1988
132. McArdle WB, Katch FI, Katch VV: Training for anaerobic and aerobic power. p. 347. In Exercise Physiology. Lea & Febiger, Philadelphia, 1986
133. McGavin CR, Gupta SP, McHardy GJR: Twelve-minute walking test for assessing disability in chronic bronchitis. BMJ 1:822, 1976
134. Cockcroft AE, Saunders MJ, Berry G: Randomised controlled trial of rehabilitation in chronic respiratory disability. Thorax 36:200, 1981
135. Dean E, Ross J, Bartz J et al: Improving the validity of exercise testing: the effect of practice on performance. Arch Phys Med Rehabil 70:599, 1989
136. Zeimetz GA, Moss RF, Butts N et al: Support versus nonsupport treadmill walking. Med Sci Sports Exerc 11:112, 1979
137. Åstrand PO, Saltin B: Maximal oxygen uptake and heart rate in various types of muscle activity. J Appl Physiol 16:977, 1961
138. Franklin BA: Exercise testing, training and arm ergometry. Sports Med 2:100, 1985
139. Sawka MN: Physiology of upper body exercise. Exerc Sport Sci Rev 14:175, 1986

140. Dean E: Assessment of the peripheral circulation: an update for practitioners. Aust J Physiother 33:164, 1987
141. Borg GAV: Perceived exertion as an indicator of somatic stress. Scand J Rehabil Med 2:92, 1970
142. Borg GAV: Psychophysiological bases of perceived exertion. Med Sci Sports Exerc 14:377, 1982
143. Eston RG, Davies BL, Williams JG: Use of perceived effort ratings to control exercise intensity in young healthy adults. Eur J Appl Physiol 56:222, 1987
144. Killian KJ, Jones NL: The use of exercise testing and other methods in the investigation of dyspnea. Clin Chest Med 5:99, 1984
145. Dean E, Ross J: Effect of walking program on patients with postpolio syndrome symptoms. Arch Phys Med Rehabil 69:1,033, 1988
146. Borg GAV, Hölmgren A, Lindbläd I: Quantitative evaluation of chest pain. Acta Med Scand 644 suppl.:S43, 1981
147. Frownfelter DL: Pulmonary rehabilitation. p. 295. In Frownfelter DL (ed): Chest Physical Therapy and Pulmonary Rehabilitation. Year Book Medical Publishers, Chicago, 1987
148. Miyashita M, Mutoh Y, Yoshioka N et al: PWC 75 percent HRmax: a measure of aerobic work capacity. Sports Med 2:159, 1985
149. Holten K: Training effect in patients with severe ventilatory failure. Scand J Resp Dis 53:65, 1972
150. Balke B, Ware RW: An experimental study of physical fitness of air force personnel. U.S. Armed Forces Med J 10:675, 1959
151. Bruce RA, Hornsten TR: Exercise stress testing in evaluation of patients with ischemic heart disease. Prog Cardiovasc Dis 11:371, 1969
152. Ellestad MH, Allen E, Wan MCK et al: Maximal treadmill stress testing for cardiovascular evaluation. Circulation 39:517, 1969
153. McHenry PL, Phillips JF, Kroebel SB: Correlation of computer-quantitated treadmill exercise electrocardiography with arteriographic localization of coronary artery disease. Am J Cardiol 30:747, 1972
154. Mason RE, Likar I: A new system of multiple-lead exercise electrocardiography. Am Heart J 71:196, 1966
155. Hellerstein HK, Horsten TR, Baker RA et al: Cardiac performance during postprandial lipemia and heparin-induced lipolysis. Am J Cardiol 20:525, 1967
156. Warring FC: Simple tests of ventilatory function used in the sanitorium and clinic. Am Rev Tuberc 60:149, 1949
157. Irwin S, Blessey RL: Patient evaluation. p. 64. In Irwin S, Tecklin JS (eds): Cardiopulmonary Physical Therapy. CV Mosby, St. Louis, 1985
158. Amon KW, Richards KL, Crawford MH: Usefulness of the postexercise response of systolic blood pressure in the diagnosis of coronary artery disease. Circulation 70:951, 1984
159. Nelson JR, Prakash C, Deedwania MD: New exercise parameter for the identification of severe coronary artery disease. Chest 95:895, 1989
160. Kappagoda CT, Greenwood PV: Physical training with minimal hospital supervision of patients after coronary artery bypass surgery. Arch Phys Med Rehabil 65:57, 1984
161. Saltin B: Physiologic adaptations to physical conditioning. Old problems revisited. Acta Med Scand 71, suppl.:S11, 1986
162. Sharkey BJ: Specificity of exercise. p. 55. In American College of Sports Medicine staff (eds): Resource Manual for Guidelines for Exercise Testing and Prescription. Lea & Febiger, Philadelphia, 1988

163. O'Hara WJ, Lasachuk, KE, Matheson PC et al: Weight training and backpacking in chronic obstuctive pulmonary disease. Respir Care 29:1,202, 1984
164. O'Hara WJ, Lasachuk KE, Matheson PC et al: Weight training benefits in chronic obstructive pulmonary disease: a controlled crossover study. Respir Care 32:660, 1987
165. Ries AL, Ellis B, Hawkins RW: Upper extremity exercise training in chronic obstructive pulmonary disease. Chest 93:688, 1988
166. Shephard RJ: Exercise and chronic lung disease. Exerc Sport Sci Rev 4:263, 1976
167. Karvonen M, Kentala K, Mustala O: The effects of training on heart rate: a longitudinal study. Annales Medicine Experimentalis et Biologiae Fenniae 35:307, 1957
168. Ward A, Malloy P, Rippe J: Exercise prescription guidelines for normal and cardiac populations. Cardiol Clin 5:197, 1987
169. Levison H, Cherniak RM: Ventilatory cost of exercise in C.O.P.D. J Appl Physiol 25:21, 1968
170. Rochester DF, Arora NS, Braun NMT et al: The respiratory muscles in chronic obstructive pulmonary disease patients. Bull Eur Physiopathol Respir 15:951, 1979
171. Mahler DA, Wells CK: Evaluation of clinical methods for rating dyspnea. Chest 93:581, 1988
172. Myles WS, Maclean D: A comparison of response and production protocols for assessing perceived exertion. Eur J Appl Physiol 55:585, 1986
173. McIlroy MB, Marshall R, Christie RV: The work of breathing in normal subjects, in mitral stenosis and emphysema. Clin Sci 13:127, 1954
174. Samsoe M: Prescription of exercise for the atypical patient with diabetes, obesity, or pulmonary disease. p. 175. In Hall LK, Meyer GC, Hellerstein HK (eds): Cardiac Rehabilitation: Exercise Testing and Prescription. SP Medical and Scientific Books, New York, 1984
175. Nickerson BG: Asthmatic patients and those with exercise-induced bronchospasm. p. 192. In Franklin BA, Gordon S, Timmis GC (eds): Exercise in Modern Medicine. Williams and Wilkins, Baltimore, 1989
176. Fitch, KD: Exercise-induced asthma and competitive athletes. Pediatrics 56, suppl.:S942, 1975.
177. deVries, HA: Healthy elderly patients. p. 215. In Franklin BA, Gordon S, Timmes GC (eds): Exercise and Modern Medicine. Williams and Wilkins, Baltimore, 1989
178. Fox EL, Matthews DK: Interval training conditioning for sports and general fitness. WB Saunders, Philadelphia, 1974
179. Nicholas JJ, Gilbert R, Gabe R et al: Evaluation of an exercise therapy program for patients with chronic obstructive pulmonary disease. Am Rev Respir Dis 102:1, 1970
180. Weiss RA, Karpovich PV: Energy cost of exercise for convalescents. Arch Phys Med July: 447, 1947

9 | Clinical Decision Making

Denise F. Patrick

The process of evaluating and treating patients with pulmonary disorders requires the physical therapist, as a clinical practitioner, to make numerous decisions throughout each day. Each decision is based on the individual's level of scientific knowledge and the experience a therapist has accumulated over time. Scientific knowledge consists of the theoretic information and physical therapy skills that a therapist is able to bring to the treatment of a patient. This knowledge/skill base allows a therapist to accumulate medical information in light of clinical observations and to begin the process of appropriate evaluation. Experience improves the therapist's ability to assimilate medical information and to set short- and long-term goals as well as determine a treatment program for each patient. Scientific knowledge and experience together provide the basis for sound clinical judgement and minimize the chance for error.

Clinical decisions are often made under time constraints. A clinician will seldom stop to consider the entire process that occurs prior to each decision. Ransden[1] has outlined the decision making process as follows:

1. *Receive:* Information arrives to the brain via vision.
2. *Infer:* Use information that is stored in memory to determine which aspect will be the focus of attention.
3. *Feel:* Respond to the information inferred.
4. *Feel about feelings:* Respond to what is felt.
5. *Determine:* What is being perceived and felt.
6. *Decide:* Prepare to take action.
7. *Act:* Carry out the decision.

The amount of time allotted to each decision may be determined by the number of patients seen within a day or clinical episodes that require an immediate response. Frequently a therapist feels these decisions are being made intuitively. Intuition, when applied to clinical decision making is a product of our theoretic knowledge and practical experience so that our course of action may intelligently be influenced.[2] The ability to make an appropriate intuitive decision requires years to develop.[3]

Physical therapy is evolving in a direction that makes physical therapists more independent.[2] The current trend toward independent practice will require physical therapy, as a profession, and the physical therapist, as an individual, to be more scientific. So much of what we use on a day to day basis has not been scientifically tested.[4] Additional research is needed to support many of the modalities and techniques currently being used. Credibility as individuals, and as a profession, will grow only if we are able to make sound clinical decisions.

This chapter discusses the characteristics and process of clinical decision making regarding the physical therapy management of pulmonary patients. This discussion is followed by three case studies to illustrate the process. Watts[4] has outlined the six characteristics involved in clinical decision making as complex, uncertain, evaluative, scientific, intuitive, and expensive. Each of these is discussed in depth below.

THE CHARACTERISTICS OF CLINICAL DECISION MAKING

Complexity

The treatment of pulmonary patients becomes complex due to the many choices to be made by the physical therapist during the process. These choices present themselves as soon as the therapist begins the evaluation process.

Assessment

One must determine which evaluative tools are necessary and safe to accurately and adequately assess the patient's clinical condition. For example, pulmonary function tests (PFTs) are helpful when diagnosing the intensity of bronchospasm during an acute asthma attack, but performing such a forceful expiratory maneuver may further increase an individual's bronchospasm. By using other less physically stressful evaluative tools such as observation and auscultation, the therapist may determine that treatment of the bronchospasm is warranted prior to the use of PFT.

Treatment

The decision making process continues on through the planning of a treatment program. An experienced therapist will be able to adequately assess evaluation results to determine if further intervention is needed. If it is, the therapist must then decide which modalities and procedures are necessary to reach specific short- and long-term goals. For example, the long-term goal of a patient referred to a pulmonary rehabilitation program may be an increase in exercise tolerance. Prior to beginning an exercise program, the patient may require a vigorous course of bronchopulmonary hygiene (BPH) to reach the short-term goal of increased airway patency, resulting in decreased resistance to airflow (sGaw) and therefore work of breathing (WOB), increased oxygenation, and decreased symptomatology of shortness of breath. Such a short-term goal involves implementation of a variety of therapeutic measures including pharmacologic management, (e.g., bronchodilators and antibiotics), postural drainage, breathing exercises, manual techniques or percussion and shaking, and a home program involving other family members to maintain pulmonary benefits. The achievement of the short-term goal will have a direct impact on the patient's ability to accomplish the long-term goal.

Treatment Modification

On occasion a therapist may determine that further treatment of a particular type is not required. A patient with advanced chronic obstructive pulmonary disease (COPD) who exhibits only a ventilatory pump limitation to exercise during a stress test may fall into such category. This can be documented by a minute ventilation ($\dot{V}e$) during the last stage of exercise that is equal to or greater than a predicted maximum voluntary ventilation (MVV). If the same test showed no indication of cardiovascular deconditioning, then an endurance program will potentially not result in any significant increase in exercise tolerance. Such a patient can benefit from breathing retraining to increase efficiency of $\dot{V}e$ and energy conservation techniques. Instruction in the use of oxygen may also be necessary if significant desaturation is observed. The decision to discontinue an endurance exercise program will require a thorough explanation to the patient, family, and physician.

Referrals

As physical therapists become more independent and specialized, the need to refer patients to another practitioner will grow.[2] Such a referral may be to a physician, another physical therapist, or other health care practitioner such as the nutritionist, social service worker, or psychiatrist. The ability to recognize when to refer is important. It is not unusual while performing a stress test on a pulmonary patient to discover signs and symptoms of cardiac disease in a patient with no previously know cardiac history. Such a situation would require appropriate referral for further diagnostic testing prior to initiating any kind of treatment program.

Discharge

Finally, the decision to discharge a patient from treatment is often complex for the therapist and difficult for the patient. If appropriate goals are initially set up then the outcome of a treatment program should reflect these goals, making the decision to discharge a patient easier.[5]

Uncertainty

The individuality of each pulmonary patient brings an element of uncertainty to the decision process for treatment. The success of any treatment program will be influenced by many factors. Patient motivation will greatly affect both the length and outcome of any treatment program. A patient recovering from abdominal or thoracic surgery who is willing to continue a program of hourly breathing exercises independently, after being properly instructed, will run a much smaller risk of postoperative pulmonary complications than the patient who remains immobile until the next treatment supervised by a therapist.

Family support, or its lack, will have a strong influence on a patient's motivation. A patient may have been the primary care giver in a family for years. With the development of a prolonged illness, such an individual may experience for the first time sympathy from other family members as well as lose some responsibilities. Fear of having to resume a former role may result in the patient ignoring any progress that is being made. A therapist may be able to recognize this when physical complaints are inconsistent with physical findings.[2] A patient who is benefitting socially from his illness or disability will want to participate in a supervised program for a much longer period of time than may be necessary. On occasion a family's being overly supportive and helpful will interfere with a patient's progress.[1] With a chronic illness such as COPD, it is very important for an individual to remain independent in activities of daily living. An overprotective family who is uncomfortable watching someone function with shortness of breath may feel a need to begin assisting the patient with various activities such as bathing and dressing. It is often difficult to make the family aware that placing the patient in a position of dependency is not beneficial.

Other factors that will have an affect on the outcome of any treatment program are the patient's emotional status, educational background, and financial status. A therapist must develop an expertise in listening to the needs of each patient and looking at the entire medical and psychosocial picture. A physical therapy program can standardize evaluation tools and documentation procedures but not patients.[3] I have found it very difficult to accurately predetermine the number of weeks a supervised outpatient pulmonary rehabilitation program should last. While some patients may be ready and willing to continue with an independent home program after 4 weeks, others will require a much longer period of time. These complicating and uncertain factors illustrate why one ''recipe'' for treating patients with a similar diagnosis will not be successful in producing change. The individuality of each patient will affect the treatment program every step of the way.

Evaluation

No one will argue about the importance of an initial evaluation and its effects on the assessment, the setting of appropriate goals, and the planning of a treatment program. This process takes on extreme importance as the physical therapist moves toward more independent practice. And yet there is a danger in allowing the process to be overdone.[2,4] Evaluation tools and techniques should be limited to those procedures that will have a direct impact on the treatment program. Carrying the procedure beyond what is necessary may be costly and discouraging to the patient. Assessing the patient's individual needs and formulating short- and long-term goals early on will help determine which evaluative procedures are necessary.

Once the initial evaluation is completed and a treatment program is in progress, there is a need for constant reassessment. Significant changes may occur during both the acute and the chronic patient's treatment. A patient being treated in the intensive care unit with bronchopulmonary hygiene may have a sudden drop in BP, requiring immediate repositioning and an increase in intravascular volume or vasopressor medications prior to continuation of the treatment. A COPD patient walking on a treadmill may have an increasing cardiac arrythmia along with a decrease in oxygen saturation (SaO_2) resulting in the need to increase oxygen flow rate so that the patient can safely continue with the exercise session. During any treatment evaluation and adjustment according to the patient's response frequently occur almost simultaneously.[4]

The development of acute symptoms in a chronically ill pulmonary patient requires reassessment of short-term goals and an adjustment in the treatment program. A COPD patient participating in an exercise program may develop an acute exacerbation due to a pulmonary infection, resulting in increased coughing, sputum production, and shortness of breath. The immediate goal would then change to clearing the infection prior to resuming the exercise program. This would require a change in medical management and an increase in treatments of BPH. Once the acute exacerbation is under control, the exercise program may be resumed. Reassessment of the patient's exercise prescription tolerance may require readjustment in the exercise prescription.

Finally, a therapist must be able to evaluate the patient's overall progress, plateau, or regression and determine which factor, such as psychosocial factors, the natural recovery or regression of the illness, or physical therapy intervention, are affecting the program. Constant reassessment is necessary until all goals have been met or the patient has plateaued.[5]

Scientific Knowledge

In combination with professional experience, scientific knowledge is the basis of our daily clinical decision making.[4] Our therapeutic choices are derived from information that is readily understood, readily recalled, and commonly encountered.[3] A therapist performing an exercise test on a patient with a well-known pulmonary history, and no known cardiac history, must be capable of recognizing cardiac symptoms. This includes the ability to interview the patient thoroughly as well as recognize the development of cardiac arrythmia, an abnormal blood pressure response to exercise, and the clinical symptoms of angina. If the patient is being treated for cardiac and pulmonary disease, the therapist must be aware of the extent of the disease, of all medications the patient is taking, and of the abnormal response to exercise that can be produced by many cardiac medications. These responses will have a great effect on the results of such an exercise test. A broad theoretical knowledge will help identify clinical symptoms.

Intuition

The role of intuition in clinical decision making combines use of the therapist's theoretical and psychosocial skills. It involves the skills of observation, listening, and communication.[2] The ability of keen observation is extremely helpful and should begin on initially meeting a patient. A COPD patient who walks into an outpatient clinic and needs to rest for several minutes, shoulders fixed and elevated, prior to communicating is someone in an advanced stage of chronic illness. Another patient using accessory muscles for tidal breathing at rest who states that shortness of breath is never experienced is someone dealing with much denial concerning his chronic disease. On a more cautious note however, we, as professionals, must not allow our initial observations to categorize patients too quickly and limit us from looking at each patient as an individual with a wide range of illness possibilities. The ability to perceive is learned: we can learn to do it better.[1]

The ability to listen will help in obtaining an accurate history from the patient. In the pulmonary population, a patient's complaints of shortness of breath, limitations in functional ability, cough, and sputum production are all significant. Being able to compare the patient's complaints with clinical observations and the results of evaluation tools will assist the therapist in determining how well educated the patient is concerning his disease, how much denial is present, and how well motivated to cooperate in recovery the patient is. A patient recovering from thoracic surgery may have continued complaints of chest wall pain and an inability to resume daily functional activities. Careful observation and palpation may reveal minimal pain and a stress test may show a normal exercise tolerance. Such a patient may lack motivation to succeed in an exercise program. A therapist's ability to recognize poor motivation as the cause for lack of progress and to relate this successfully to the patient and family are the result of effective psychosocial skills. The development of such skills will allow a master clinician to meet the many needs of each patient, to relate to patients on their level and to communicate to patients' families and other health care providers.[4,5]

Expense

Although an individual physical therapy session is not costly, a prolonged rehabilitation program is.[4] A therapist involved in independent practice or practice without referral must be careful not to overtreat or allow patients to stay in a program longer than is necessary. Many third party payors have set very specific guidelines as to what will or will not be reimbursed. Documentation of what we do and how we do it is our only means of proving these guidelines are reasonable or not reasonable and that guidelines are being observed if appropriate for a given patient. We must become skilled at stating a specific problem, setting a goal to alleviate the problem, and determining a treatment program to reach the goal. To ensure our continued financial success, our documentation must be meaningful, accurate, and performed immediately and systematically.[6]

THE PROCESS OF CLINICAL DECISION MAKING

The comprehensive treatment of pulmonary patients can be broken down into four categories of treatment:

1. *Breathing retraining*
   Muscles of ventilation
   Positions of relaxation
   Improved breathing patterns at rest and with activity
   Inspiratory muscle training
   Education
2. *Bronchopulmonary hygiene*
   Proper use of medication
   Hydration
   Secretion clearance
   Home program
   Education
3. *Posture/muscle imbalances*
   Exercises for flexibility
   Exercises for muscle strengthening
   Exercises to maintain or improve posture
   Home program
   Education
4. *Endurance training*
   Walking, jogging, or bicycling program
   Home program
   Education

The individual needs of each patient will require emphasis on specific components of each category. A treatment program for an acutely ill patient in an intensive care unit having difficult weaning from a ventilator may emphasize breathing retraining and bronchopulmonary hygiene. A few months later the treatment program for the same patient, being seen in an outpatient clinic due to decreased functional ability, may emphasize exercise programs for posture, increased muscle strength, and endurance. Other patients may require various components from all four categories at any given time. Since no two patients have an identical clinical presentation, it is essential that treatment programs be individualized. The decision making model as outlined by Holden[5] in Figure 9-1 is an effective mechanism for avoiding delivery of routine care.

Patient–Therapist Interaction

The arrows between the patient and therapist signify the constant interaction that is affected by the skills of the therapist and the needs of the patient. The key decisions made by the therapist are located in the middle of the diagram and comprise the decision making process. The boxes on the outside represent all the factors that influence the outcome of the decision making process.

The Patient's View

For the patient these factors are physical problems and psychosocial status. Although a therapist must be aware of the patient's entire medical history, the emphasis of treatment will be directed to those specific problems that resulted in

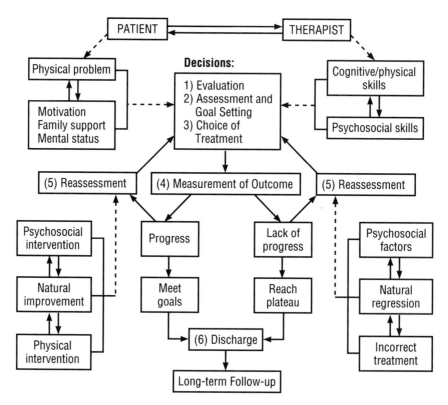

Fig. 9-1. Flow chart illustrating the decision making model.

the patient seeking the assistance of a physical therapist. The major psychosocial factors that will affect the patient's decision making process are motivation, family support, and mental status.

The Therapist's View

On the part of the therapist, the factors that will affect the outcome of the decision making process are cognitive/physical skills and psychosocial skills. In order to avoid making errors during clinical decision making, a therapist must have a thorough understanding of the patient's medical problems and knowledge of the means available for treatment. Enough emphasis cannot be placed on the importance of the therapist's ability to communicate to a patient and his family on their level. The therapist must listen to the day to day needs of the individual patient to avoid setting goals that the patient has no interest in achieving.

How Decisions Are Made

The decision making process follows six stages:

1. Evaluation
2. Assessment and goal setting
3. Choice of treatment
4. Measurement of outcome
5. Reassessment
6. Discharge

The complete evaluation process includes review of history, patient interview, choice of evaluation tools, and performance of evaluation. Once the evaluation is completed the therapist will be able to prioritize the clinical problems requiring further intervention and begin to set short- and long-term goals for the entire treatment program. Each clinical problem will require a treatment plan. If clinical problems have been prioritized appropriately, then achieving short-term goals will ready the patient for whatever tasks have been set to achieve long-term goals. Documentation of the patient's status on a regular basis will help measure the outcome of a treatment program and determine whether the goals are being met. If goals are not being met, a reassessment will determine why. Possible causes for lack of improvement are (1) the natural progression or regression of the acute or chronic illness, (2) an acute change in the medical status of the patient, (3) intervening psychosocial factors of the patient, and (4) the need to change the present treatment program. Reassessment continues until the goals have been met or the patient reaches a plateau and is no longer responding to treatment. The decision to discontinue therapy should be relatively easy at this point.

The decision making process is illustrated in the following three case studies.

CASE STUDY # 1

The patient is a 54-year-old woman who presented herself to a walk-in clinic with the chief complaint of swelling in both lower extremities for the past 10 days. She admitted to a smoking history of one pack per day for 40 years, had no complaint of shortness of breath or cough, and had not seen a physician in 20 years. Examination for deep venous thrombosis was negative. The most significant finding of all other lab work was a hematocrit of 58.7. A room air arterial blood gas was then drawn, resulting in a PaO_2 of 42 mmHg, $PaCO_2$ of 62 mmHg, and pH of 7.38. A ventilation perfusion scan was negative for pulmonary embolus. It was decided that she would be admitted to the hospital for further evaluation and treatment.

Physical examination revealed a thin, cyanotic-appearing female. Her skin was mottled and her extremities were purplish with blanching. Heart sounds included an S1, S2, and loud S3. The lungs had decreased breath sounds throughout with no rales or rhonchi. The lower extremities were observed to have 3+ pitting edema to the midcalf and 1+ to the thigh.

Further evaluation revealed the following significant results:

Chest X-ray. Her chest x-ray was consistent with COPD with hyperinflation, flat diaphragms, narrowing of smaller lung vessels, and prominence of the central pulmonary artery; the heart was moderately enlarged and there was no evidence of congestive heart failure or infiltrates.

Pulmonary Function Tests. The results of her tests (see Table 9-1) represented significant obstructive disease.

Electrocardiogram. The electrocardiogram (ECG) revealed sinus tachycardia at 100 bpm; leads 2, 3, and F were with an enlarged P wave, inverted T wave, and a Q wave.

Echocardiogram. The echocardiogram showed right ventricular hypertrophy and enlargement; there was moderate hypokinesis, some excess pericardial fluid, but excellent left ventricular function.

Table 9-1. Pulmonary Function Test for Case Study #1

Test	Actual Measure	Percent of Predicted Measure
Forced vital capacity (FVC)	1.5 L	42
Forced expiratory volume for one second (FEV_1)	.4 L	15
Ratio of FEV_1: FVC	27%	36
Residual volume (RV)	4.35 L	225
Functional residual volume (FRV)	5.09 L	163
Total lung capacity (TLC)	6.15 L	110
Ratio of RY:TLC	74%	206
Midmaximal flow rate (MMF)	.125 L	4
Diffusion capacity (DLCO)	9.5 L	44

Diagnosis. She was diagnosed as having severe COPD with hypoxemia, hypercapnia, polycthemia, and cor pulmonale.

The first major concern was careful correction of hypoxemia and hypercapnia. Initially she was placed on .5 L of O_2 via nasal cannula. This resulted in an arterial blood gas (ABG) of 49/58/7.38 (values: PaO_2, $PaCO_2$, pH). Gradually the oxygen flow was increased to 1.5 L with a corresponding arterial blood gas of 55/57/7.39. SaO_2 levels were monitored closely and it was found that the patient required 3 L O_2 during low level activity (such as ambulation to the bathroom) to maintain an SaO_2 above 85 percent with exercise. Other medications included intravenous Aminophylline and Solu-Medrol, beginning at 60 mg. She was also given an inhaled bronchodialator albuterol, via a micronebulizer. She was phlebotomized because of the initial hemotcrit of 58.7, which improved to 50. As her oxygenation improved she diuresed spontaneously and lost 14 pounds. Her right sided heart failure did not require any further diuresing during the hospital admission.

The patient was discharged to home on the seventh day. A liquid oxygen system was delivered to her house and she was instructed to use it 24 hours per day at 1.5 L during rest and 3 L with any activity. Her medications included Theo-Dur, 300 mg bid; an Alupent inhaler, two puffs q4h; and Prednisone, 40 mg qd, that would be tapered over the next few weeks. The patient was to be followed closely by internal and pulmonary medicine. She was also referred to chest physical therapy for an outpatient pulmonary rehabilitation program.

Evaluation

Observation. All of the information presented thus far was available to the therapist prior to the patient's initial visit in the outpatient physical therapy department. The initial clinic visit was scheduled 5 days after her discharge from the hospital. On that day she arrived carrying a portable oxygen tank set at 3 L. She presented as very thin and cachetic, appearing older than her stated age. Her posture was with fixed, elevated shoulders and her breathing pattern incorporated mild use of accessory muscles with a prolonged expiratory phase and RR of 20.

After several minutes of resting her breathing pattern improved to upper chest expansion with some diaphragmatic expansion at the end of the inspiratory phase. Her preferred sitting posture was leaning forward, supporting her upper extremities with elbows extended on her thighs.

Patient Interview. The patient was initially quite noncommunicative. She answered all questions with very brief statements and her only question in return was whether or not her need for oxygen was permanent. She essentially had no complaints of shortness of breath, cough or sputum production. She did admit to having noticed some increased fatigue for the month previous to her hospital admission. Since her discharge she had managed to perform all of her personal activities of daily living.

She was divorced and living at home with three sons all above 21. Up until her hospital admission she had performed all household chores. She stated her sons had helped some since her return home. The only stairs she needed to climb were down and up from the basement to do laundry. She had not attempted this or any other housework since her discharge from the hospital.

She was employed as a secretary for a local school. Due to her long-term employment there, arrangements had been made for her not to return to work for several months. She did not tell her employer that she would be returning with portable oxygen.

Since her discharge she had continued not to smoke cigarettes and had been using her oxygen 24 hours per day at 1.5 L during rest and 3 L with any activity.

Physical Examination. Her BP at rest was 122/86, HR was 83 beats per minute (bpm), RR was 16 and SaO_2 was 95 percent on 1.5 L O_2. Physical characteristics that were representative of long standing lung disease were as follows: inspiratory to expiratory ratio of 1:1.5, increased anterior posterior to lateral diameter of 1:1, subcostal angle of 110 degrees; posterior excursion was absent. Breath sounds were with markedly decreased air movement; no rales or rhonchi were heard. There was 1+ pitting edema of both ankles. In a supine position she was able to improve diaphragmatic expansion with relaxation and much verbal and tactile stimulation. It was decided that she would benefit from a pulmonary rehabilitation program and that further evaluation would continue on subsequent clinic visits to include posture, strength, range of motion, and exercise testing.

Posture evaluation revealed minimal thoracic deformities: supraclavicular retraction was present, the sternum slightly protruded, and right shoulder and hip were slightly higher than left, with a small lumbar scoliosis. Range of motion was within normal limits for all extremities, as were forward and lateral trunk flexion. There was some limitation in trunk extension and rotation. Strength of upper and lower abdominals was fair. Strength of all other muscle groups was good. Evaluation of all the above was performed using 3 L O_2 and frequent rest periods. The patient was clinically observed to demonstrate respiratory distress during minimal activity by an increased respiratory rate to 24, increased use of accessory muscles, and an increased HR to 120 bpm. SaO_2 remained above 90 percent. Despite all of the above clinical observations, she did not subjectively complain of shortness of breath.

Testing

On her third clinic visit an exercise test was performed on a stationary bicycle (see Table 9-2). The test was performed in 6-minute stages with a rest period between stages. She was able to complete two full stages of

Table 9-2. Results of Exercise Test for Case Study #1

Stage	Time (minutes)	HR (beats per minute)[a]	BP	RR	SaO$_2$ (%)	Comments
Resting		117	130/80	18	94	
Stage 1						Patient was very nervous about exercising. At the end of stage 1 she complained of leg fatigue but no shortness of breath.
.25 KP	2	120	130/80	20	94	
30 rpm	4	111	130/80	20	94	
7.5 W	6	114	130/80	20	93	
	1 p̄	115	130/80	16	94	
Stage 2						At the end of stage 2 she complained of overall fatigue but still no shortness of breath. She was able to maintain a coordinated breathing pattern with significant increase in her work of breathing.
.5 KP	2	129	130/80	18	95	
40 rpm	4	131	140/92	18	94	
22 W	6	142	136/80	24	92	
	1 p̄	119	142/86	16	93	
Posttest	2 p̄	102	130/80	12	96	

Abbreviations: HR, heart rate; BP, blood pressure; RR, respiratory rate; SaO$_2$, oxygen saturation; KP, kiloponds; rpm, revolutions per minute; W, watts; p̄, posttest.

[a] Predicted maximum heart rate was 166 beats per minute.

exercise. Because of her need for oxygen we were unable to collect accurate expired gases and therefore unable to determine a $\dot{V}e$ for maximum exercise. She did exhibit normal BP and HR response to exercise and no cardiac arrythmia was observed. She was able to reach 85 percent of a predicted maximum HR, but this was done at a very low workload of 20 watts (W). She was able to maintain a coordinated breathing pattern throughout, but a significant increase in her WOB was observed during the last 2 minutes of exercise. SaO_2 remained adequate throughout the test on 3 L O_2.

The interpretation of the exercise test documentated that she exhibited primarily a pulmonary limitation to exercise with some cardiovascular deconditioning. Her predicted MVV was only 14 L/min. Although we were unable to obtain a $\dot{V}e$ at maximum exercise, it was assumed that with an RR of 24 and a forced expiratory volume in 1 second (FEV_1) of .4 L she had reached her predicted MVV. Her high HR at such a low work load can be interpreted as cardiovascular deconditioning, as can her complaint of leg fatigue.

Assessment and Goals

The entire evaluation process occurred over three separate clinic visits. The therapist was able to begin assessing the clinical problem that required further intervention during the first session. Table 9-3 lists the clinical problems, in the order in which the therapist felt they needed to be addressed, along with the short- and long-term goals and a treatment plan for each. It is important to emphasize that both the treatment and the home program were initiated at the time of the first clinic visit. During this session the patient was instructed in the mechanics of normal ventilation and respiration and the changes that occur with COPD, the importance of relaxation as a technique, various positions to be used during episodes of stress, and controlled diaphragmatic breathing in a resting position. She was asked to practice diaphragmatic breathing at home and to begin incorporating the other techniques into her day to day life. Energy conservation tactics such as exhalation on effort and controlled breathing patterns during walking, stair climbing, and other activities of daily living were added during the second clinic visit. The patient was also made aware of the clinical symptoms of increased respiratory distress, such as an increase in WOB, RR, and HR, that may occur with rest or minimal activity. The therapist felt this was an important step in the processes of increasing the patient's awareness of her chronic disease, accepting of her need of oxygen, and dealing with her denial.

The patient was seen on an individual basis for three initial clinic visits. The results of the exercise test indicated that the patient would tolerate and benefit from continued participation in a rehabilitation program that included endurance training. This required a commitment on the part of the

Table 9-3. Clinical Problems and Treatment Plan for Case Study #1

Clinical Problems	Treatment Plan
Abnormal breathing pattern STG: improve diaphragmatic breathing at rest LTG: control breathing pattern with activity	Education: mechanics of breathing and chronic changes that occur with COPD Breathing exercises in supine Paced breathing with walking Position of relaxation
Increased work of breathing with low level activity STG: decrease use of accessory muscles LTG: increase use of diaphragm	Education: disease process, oxygen, medications Energy conservation techniques Controlled breathing patterns

Denial
STG: acceptance and use of oxygen,
  recognition of dyspnea
LTG: understanding of chronic disease,
  continue not smoking
	Emotional support
	Referral to psychiatrist if indicated

Posture STG: maintain present posture LTG: improve muscle strength	Flexibility exercises Strengthening exercises

Deconditioning
STG: interval training program
LTG: 20 consecutive minutes of exercise,
  independent home program
	Education: need for long-term compliance
	Endurance exercise program on a stationary
	  bicycle

Abbreviations: STG, short-term goals; LTG, long-term goals; COPD, chronic obstructive pulmonary disease.

patient to three clinic visits per week for a minimum of 6 weeks. Ultimately 10 weeks were necessary to reach the final goal of an independent home program. Continued reassessment and adjustment of the treatment plan was necessary throughout the 10-week period. We will now look at this more closely.

Treatment, Measurement of Outcome, and Reassessment

Week One

The patient was instructed in a list of exercises emphasizing thoracic flexibility and strengthening of upper extremities, back, and abdominal muscle groups. These exercises were performed with controlled breathing patterns and exhalation on effort principles. They were used as warm-up exercise prior to use of the bicycle ergometer and incorporated into her home program.

A stationary bicycle was chosen for her endurance exercise program for several reasons. A controlled environment avoiding the extreme temperature and weather changes common to New England was necessary with her COPD. The patient chose to perform her exercise program on a long-term basis within the privacy of her own home. By raising the bike handlebars she was able to lean forward and support herself with her upper extremities, stabilizing the accessory muscles and allowing her to concentrate on maximizing the function of the diaphragm and eliminating the need to carry her oxygen.

During each exercise session she was monitored for BP, HR, RR, and SaO_2. Breathing patterns were constantly observed and corrected when necessary. For the first week, a two lead telemetry unit monitored her electrocardiogram. This was discontinued because no arrythmia was observed.

Her initial exercise prescription was established as follows: an intensity of 20 W and a duration of 4 minutes of cycling alternating with 2 minutes of rest for 16 minutes of total cycling time, performed 3 times per week.

Measurement of Outcome.   Cycling time was limited to 4-minute segments due to an increased RR from 16 to 24 and a desaturation from 96 to 88 percent. After 2 minutes of rest the RR returned to 16 and the SaO_2 to 97 percent. She continued to use 1.5 L O_2 at rest and 3 L with activity. Although objectively a significant increase in her WOB was noted whenever her RR approached 24, she subjectively continued not to complain of shortness of breath. She did remain nervous about exercising.

Reassessment.   The exercise prescription required alteration during the second exercise session due to an increase in RR to 24 and a desaturation to 85 percent after only 3 minutes of cycling. One difference noted in her medical management was that her steroid program had been tapered to an every other day regimen. The second exercise session occurred on a day without steroids. Subjectively, the patient did not perceive this day as more difficult. The exercise prescription was changed to a duration of 3 minutes cycling alternating with 2 minutes of rest, for a total exercise time of 12 minutes.

Week Two

The patient continued to experience increased respiratory distress by observation on the days she did not take steroids. Subjectively, she began to notice that these days were symptomatically more difficult. Her physician was contacted and the steroids were increased to 20 mg daily for 3 days. On the fourth day she was to decrease the steroids to 10 mg and begin using an Azmacort Inhaler for 2 puffs tid.

Measurement of Outcome.   Although there was no change in her pulmonary function (FEV_1 remained at .4 L) with the increased steroids, clinically she was able to perform more exercise with a lower RR and HR and a higher SaO_2. The patient began to subjectively perceive dyspnea.

Reassessment.   The duration of the exercise prescription was increased to 6 minutes of cycling alternating with 2 minutes of rest, for total cycling time of 24 minutes. She was also instructed to use the Alupent Inhaler prior to each exercise session.

Week Three

She continued to feel well on daily doses of steroids. The 10 mg of steroid were extended for 3 days because she forgot to initiate the inhaled steroid as instructed.

Measurement of Outcome. During exercise sessions she was able to maintain SaO_2 levels above 94 percent, a maximum RR of 20 and a maximum HR of 120 bpm.

Reassessment. The duration of the exercise prescription was increased to 8 minutes of cycling alternating with 2 minutes of rest, for a total cycling time of 24 minutes.

Week Four

On Monday oral steroids were discontinued. Despite the continued use of the inhaled steroids the patient arrived on Friday with complaints of increased respiratory distress and increased cough and sputum production.

Measurement of Outcome. On Friday the exercise session was terminated after 5 minutes of cycling due to a BP of 148/86, an HR of 128, an RR of 30 and an SaO_2 below 90 percent. PFT values remained unchanged with a FEV_1 of .4 L and a forced vital capacity (FVC) of 2 L.

Reassessment. Her physician was once again contacted. She was instructed to continue with the Azmacort Inhaler and to add 20 mg of oral steroid every other day. Both the physician and the therapist felt that she obtained a consistent significant increase in functional capacity on low levels of steroids.

Week Five

The patient was now able to recognize that subjectively she felt better on the days that she was taking steroids. She continued to complain of an increased cough and sputum production as well as a change in the color of the sputum.

Measurement of Outcome. A sputum sample was sent to microbiology. At the end of the week her symptoms continued to worsen and her respiratory distress increased. At rest her RR was 20 and her HR was 119. Her temperature remained afebrile.

Reassessment. At the beginning of the week the duration of the exercise prescription was decreased to 5 minutes of cycling alternating with 3 minutes of rest, for a total exercise time of 20 minutes. She was instructed to increase the use of her bronchodilator and steroid inhaler to every 3 hours on the days she did not take any oral steroids. She was started on an antibiotic (Bactrim) and treated with BPH during her clinic visit at the end of the week.

Week Six

The results of the sputum sample did not show any acute infection, but the patient continued with increased respiratory distress.

Measurement of Outcome. PFT results deteriorated to an FVC of .9 L and an FEV_1 of .3 L. Her ankles demonstrated an increase in edema, and during exercise, SaO_2 decreased to 81 percent, with an HR of 140 bpm and an RR of 24.

Reassessment. The oxygen flow rate was increased to 4 L to maintain an SaO_2 above 85 percent for the remainder of the exercise session. Steriods were once again increased to 20 mg daily and remained at that level for the duration of the rehabilitation program. Lasix was added to her medical management at 20 mg daily. The exercise prescription remained unchanged.

Week Seven

All of the acute symptoms of increased respiratory distress (shortness of breath, cough, and sputum production) improved.

Measurement of Outcome. The patient was able to exercise with a maximum BP of 130/82, a maximum HR of 120 bpm, a maximum RR of 24, and an SaO_2 that remained above 90 percent on 3 L O_2 via nasal prongs.

Reassessment. The duration of the exercise prescription was advanced to 7 minutes of cycling alternating with 1 minute of rest, for a total of 21 minutes of cycling.

Weeks Eight and Nine

The patient was now able to identify a good day from a bad day, as well as various factors that had a specific effect, such as hot, humid weather and proper use of all her medications. She purchased a stationary bicycle for home use and began using it every day that she did not come to the clinic.

Measurement of Outcome. All vital signs were within good limits during each exercise session. SaO_2 remained above 92 percent on 3 L O_2.

Reassessment. The duration of exercise prescription advanced to 25 minutes of cycling with only 1 minute of rest after 10 minutes.

Week Ten

Subjectively, the patient felt more energetic for the rest of the day if she exercised early in the morning.

Measurement of Outcome.   The patient was able to maintain an SaO_2 above 90 percent while exercising with 2 L O_2.

Reassessment.   The final exercise prescription was as follows: an intensity of 25 W, a duration of 20 to 25 consecutive minutes, and a frequency of 5 to 7 times per week. Both the therapist and the patient felt she was ready to continue this above program independently at home.

Discharge

The patient returned to the outpatient clinic 4 weeks later for a reassessment of the home program. At that time her medications consisted of Theo-Dur, 300 mg bid; Alupent inhaler, 2 puffs qid; Prednisone, 20 mg qd; and Lasix, 40 mg qd. She continued to use the Alupent inhaler prior to each exercise session.

Referring back to the list of clinical problems, the therapist felt that most of the short- and long-term goals had been met. At rest, the patient's RR was 12, and with most activities she was using a pursed lip breathing pattern and maintaining an RR below 20. She continued to have mild use of her accessory muscles at all times but posterior excursion had increased to 1 inch.

This patient was able to continue not to smoke. She was functioning at a satisfactory level by having made certain compromises such as having the groceries delivered to home from the supermarket and not carrying the laundry back upstairs. She continued to use her oxygen 24 hours a day at 1.5 L at rest and at 2 L with activity. Her plans were to return to her secretarial job within 2 months. It was felt that all the goals concerning the patient's initial denial of her chronic disease had been met and further intervention was not needed at this time.

She had maintained excellent motivation for her home exercise program and was using her stationary bicycle for 25 to 30 minutes daily. Each session was preceded and followed by the flexibility and strengthening exercises as warm-up/cool-down periods. She tolerated 25 minutes of exercise with a maximum BP of 150/96, a maximum HR of 128 bpm, a maximum RR of 18, and an SaO_2 that remained above 88 percent with 2 L O_2. Her pulmonary function remained unchanged compared to 4 months earlier. The therapist and the patient felt that she was functioning at a satisfactory level and that she remained well motivated to continue the home program independently.

Of interest is that 6 weeks after her discharge from the pulmonary rehabilitation program, her physician once again tapered her use of steroids and this time was more successful. Within 4 weeks she was maintained on 20 mg of Prednisone every other day along with the Azmacort Inhaler, 2 puffs qid. She was also no longer requiring Lasix on a daily basis and had returned to work full time.

CASE STUDY # 2

The patient is a 71-year-old woman who was admitted for elective surgery on February 5 to resect a transverse arch aneurysm. Her major complaint at that time was increasing shortness of breath for the past 6 months. The aneurysm was discovered on routine chest x-ray and confirmed by CT scan.

The patient had a significant past medical history that placed her in a high risk category for surgery and included ploycystic kidney disease, COPD, and hypertension. She had a 35-year history of chronic renal failure with a baseline creatinine of 5 and a blood ureanitrogen (BUN) of 70. Although she had stopped smoking 4 years prior to this surgery she did have a 75 pack-year smoking history. The hypertension was being treated with nadolol (Corgard) and furosemide (Lasix). Her BP at rest was 160/85. Her complaints were shortness of breath with minimal activity, and occasional productive cough, two-pillow orthopnea, and hoarseness for the past 2 years. She wore a hearing aide for decreased auditory acuity.

Pre-operative evaluation revealed the following:

Chest X-ray. The aorta showed a localized dilation of its ascending portion, upward and to the left, consistent with a vascular aneurysm of the ascending aorta. The left diaphragm was markedly elevated, suggesting the possibility of nerve involvement. There was mild left ventricular enlargement. No infiltrates or atelectasis were seen. The costophrenic angles were clear and there was no evidence of effusion.

Computed Tomography Scan. A six cm aneurysm of the ascending aorta was confirmed by computed tomography (CT).

Exercise Test with Thallium. The patient was able to complete 7 minutes of the Bruce Protocol. The test was terminated because of shortness of breath. She was able to reach only 67 percent of her predicted maximum HR, which indicated a low physical work capacity. The ECG remained in normal sinus rhythm, with occasional premature ventricular contractions during exercise and rare premature atrial contractions during recovery. There were no ischemic ECG changes observed throughout the test and she had no complaints representing angina. She did exhibit a slight decrease in BP at peak exercise. Mild left ventricular dysfunction was observed but there were no pulmonary perfusion defects.

Pulmonary Function Tests. In PFTs, her forced vital capacity (FVC) was 1.6 L (52 percent of predicted) and the FEV_1 was 1.1 L (48 percent of predicted).

Renal Consult. Patients with polycystic kidney disease tend to have an increased incidence of cerebral aneurysm when compared to the general population. Because of this, an MRI (magnetic resonance image) was taken of her brain that revealed lacunar infarcts of the thalamus and left cerebral hemisphere.

Verapamil was added to the management of her hypertension to bring her BP down to 130 to 140/80. This decrease in BP would potentially reduce or slow down the rate of progression of her kidney disease in the postoperative period.

Maintaining adequate fluid balance was also very important. Normal saline was to begin 24 hours prior to surgery and continue throughout. This was to be accompanied by Lasix just prior to the induction of anesthesia.

Assessment and Goals

A pre-operative exam by physical therapy revealed breath sounds with decreased aeration throughout both lung fields and an occasional inspiratory wheeze that was not reproducible with every breath. Her RR was 16 and her breathing pattern at rest was predominantly upper chest expansion. Any attempt at maximal inspiration required the use of accessory muscles. She had poor chest wall mobility and poor diaphragmatic excursion. Her cough was tight and raspy but nonproductive prior to surgery.

Table 9-4 represents the clinical problems, goals, and treatment plan for this patient throughout the remainder of her hospital stay. Prior to surgery the short-term goals were (1) to improve breathing patterns and diaphragmatic expansion, (2) to have the patient develop an understanding of the need for postoperative pulmonary care in preventing complications, (3) to instruct the patient in techniques of bed mobility and coughing with splinting, (4) to introduce the patient to manual techniques of percussion and shaking, and (5) to develop the patient's confidence and willingness to cooperate in the postoperative period. Long-term goals were to prevent postoperative pulmonary complications and have the patient return to her present functional level.

Treatment, Measurement of Outcome, and Reassessment

On February 13 she underwent repair of the aneurysm with a Dacron patch. The cardiopulmonary bypass time was 120 minutes, with 35 minutes of cross-clamp time. Throughout the procedure she received 3 L of normal saline, 4 units of red blood cells, 4 units of fresh frozen cells, and 30 units of platelets. There were no major complications and she was brought to the intensive care unit (ICU) intubated and ventilated in stable condition.

Her cardiac output ($\dot{Q}$) was 3.8 L, ECG was in normal sinus rhythm at 70, and her BP was 100/80. Chest x-ray demonstrated some evidence of volume overload, but no cardiomegaly, pneumothorax, or infiltrates were seen. She was being ventilated with a tidal volume (Vt) of 800 cc, intermittent mandatory ventilation (IMV) of 8 and a fraction of inspired oxygen (FiO_2) of 50 percent. ABG values were 102/38/7.35 (values: PaO_2, $PaCO_2$, pH).

Table 9-4. Clinical Problems and Treatment Plan for Case Study #2

Clinical Problems	Treatment Plan
Pre-operative period	
STG: decrease work of breathing and increase ventilation, develop patient's confidence and her understanding of need for post operative pulmonary care	Education: BPH, bed mobility, coughing, tubes and lines, pain medication
	Improve breathing pattern with breathing exercises
LTG: prevent post operative pulmonary complications, improve functional level	BPH
	Exercise program
Immediate post operative period	
STG: mobilize secretions, increase ventilation, decrease work of breathing, decrease $\dot{V}_A:\dot{Q}$ mismatch	BPH: manual techniques, suctioning, hyperinflation, positioning
	Wean from ventilator
LTG: independent breathing	
Failure to wean	
STG: mobilize secretions, increase ventilation, decrease $\dot{V}_A:\dot{Q}$ mismatch, clear pneumonia, decrease work of breathing and protect upper airway, increase mobility and strength, decrease volume, improve nutrition	BPH and inhaled bronchodilators
	Antibiotics and BPH
	Tracheostomy
	Low level exercise program: transfers and ambulation
	Diuresis and chest tube
LTG: wean from ventilator, improve ventilatory mechanics	Gastrostomy tube
	Decrease IMV, increase time on t-piece, ventilatory muscle training, nocturnal positive pressure
	Diaphragmatic plication
Weaned	
STG: mobilize secretions and decrease work of breathing, increase strength and endurance	Remains in place, BPH by nursing staff
	Range of motion exercises, ambulation, cycle ergometer endurance program
LTG: discharge from hospital	Home program

Abbreviations: STG, short-term goals; LTG, long-term goals; $\dot{V}_A:\dot{Q}$, ratio of alveolar ventilation to perfusion; BPH, bronchopulmonary hygiene; IMV, intermittent mandatory ventilation.

First Postoperative Day

The major concerns for the immediate postoperative period were her hemodynamic status, renal function, and respiratory management. Hemodynamically, the goals were to avoid hypertension and watch closely for bleeding. Systolic blood pressure (SBP) was to be kept under 140 and she would be transfused with platelets if her hematocrit dropped below 20. Her chronic renal failure placed her at high risk for volume overload. It was important to watch her potassium (K) and bicarbonate (HCO_3) levels closely and maintain an adequate urine output with Lasix. Respiratory management involved keeping the patient sedated and ventilated overnight.

Measurement of Outcome. On the first postoperative day the patient remained intubated and vented on an IMV of 8. She was awake and able to nod appropriately to questions but she did not demonstrate any spontaneous breathing. Breath sounds were markedly diminished, primarily at her left base, but there was no wheezing. She was afebrile, her BP was

120/60, her HR was 102 bpm, and her ABG was 166/34/7.32. One concern was the drainage from her chest tube, which had already been over 2 L. Another major concern was the transection of the left phrenic, recurrent laryngeal, and vagus nerves, which occurred during the surgery, resulting in paralysis of the left diaphragm and vocal cords.

Reassessment. The patient was determined to be hemodynamically stable for treatment but it was felt that vigorous manual techniques of percussion and shaking should be avoided due to the increased drainage from the chest tube site. She was treated with postural drainage, breathing exercises with a hyperinflation bag, gentle vibration to her chest wall, and suctioning via the endotracheal tube to stimulate coughing, clear secretions, and improve ventilation. Suctioning produced a minimal amount of bloody secretions. At the end of treatment she was placed in a right semi-prone position to promote expansion of the left lung. She remained stable throughout the treatment with a chest tube drainage of 210 cc. There was a significant increase in aeration posttreatment primarily at the bases. The treatments were repeated every 4 hours. The short-term goals were to prevent acute postoperative pulmonary complications and begin weaning the patient from the ventilator. The long-term goal was independent spontaneous breathing.

Second Postoperative Day

Measurement of Outcome. The patient remained hemodynamically stable and the process of weaning her from the ventilator was started by gradually decreasing the IMV rate to 4. Concomitantly, the patient was spontaneously breathing at a rate of 16. ABG values were 147/43/7.28. Her breath sounds included increased wheezing throughout, and a larger amount of secretions were obtained with suctioning. Unfortunately the patient extubated herself. Initially, with a face mask set at 60 percent O_2, her ABG was 171/41/7.30. Her RR was 20 and her breathing pattern was labored.

Reassessment. Treatment of BPH continued, with the addition of oral bronchodilators (.5 cc albuterol [Ventolin] with 1.5 cc normal saline) via a hand held micronebulizer. Her cough was weak and ineffective. She continued to require suctioning for secretion clearance, which now needed to be done via her nasotracheal passage.

Third Postoperative Day

Measurement of Outcome. Hemodynamically, she remained stable, with a maximum BP of 140/80 and an HR between 80 and 100 bpm in normal sinus rhythm. Her BUN and creatinine remained at baseline and her urine output was satisfactory. Her weight was up 3.4 kg from her pre-operative weight. Her pulmonary status began to deteriorate. Over the next few days the patient became very lethargic. Her RR was 24 and she exhibited a discoordinated breathing pattern. Her temperature spiked to 100.2 degrees, breath sounds were with diffuse expiratory wheezes, and there was a further increase in sputum production. On the fifth postoperative day (February 18), chest x-ray revealed a left lower lobe pneumonia. Her white blood count increased to 20.5 and a sputum culture was positive for *Pseudomonas aeruginosa*. Her ABG values deteriorated to 59/50/7.25 while she wore a face mask delivering 100 percent O_2.

Reassessment. She was started on intravenous (IV) antibiotics of gentamicin and ceftazidime for treatment of the pneumonia. In response to the decreasing O_2 and increasing CO_2 she was reintubated and ventilated. Physical therapy treatments continued to emphasize vigorous BPH and included oral bronchodilators, postural drainage, manual techniques, hyperinflation, and suctioning. The short-term goal was now to clear the pneumonia, and the long-term goal was to wean the patient from the ventilator.

Failure to Wean

Measurement of Outcome. Although the patient was extubated on February 25, following a slow weaning process, she again failed due to poor respiratory reserve. Her RR at rest was 30, with a discoordinated breathing pattern. Pulmonary mechanics were an inspiratory force of −35 mmHg, Vt of 250 ml, and a VC of 400 to 500 ml. Secretions and mucus plugging, along with an ineffective cough, remained a constant problem. Her ECG showed occasional premature atrial and ventricular contractions as well as runs of bigeminy. On March 3, due to mental status changes and an ABG of 75/45/7.31 on 100 percent face mask plus 4 L/min O_2 via nasal prongs, she was reintubated.

Reassessment. While the patient was extubated BPH had continued to be the most important element of her treatment plan. In addition, a low level activity program was started to include ambulation. At rest oxygen was provided via a 100 percent face mask. During ambulation nasal prongs were utilized. SaO_2 levels at rest were 96 percent on 4 L/min oxygen. During ambulation the oxygen was increased to 6 L/min. After ambulating 10 feet, her SaO_2 level decreased to 93 percent and her RR increased to 40. The patient needed maximal assistance for all transfers and ambulation. Shortly after reintubation she underwent a tracheostomy to protect her upper airway, assist in management of secretions, and decrease her WOB.

After the Tracheostomy

Measurement of Outcome. The patient remained dependent on ventilatory support till the middle of May. Numerous factors contributed to her inability to wean:

1. sputum cultures still positive for pseudomonas aeruginosa
2. a white blood cell count (WBC) of 23.6
3. copious secretions and mucous plugging
4. fluid overload with a 2.7 kg increase in weight
5. a right pleural effusion requiring drainage with a chest tube
6. underlying COPD
7. left hemidiaphragm paralysis
8. poor nutritional status
9. a hematocrit of 33.6

Reassessment. Short-term goals were to: (1) constantly mobilize secretions, (2) improve ventilation, (3) decrease alveolar ventilation to perfusion ($\dot{V}_A:\dot{Q}$) mismatch, (4) decrease the WOB, and (5) maintain mobility and muscle strength. Treatment emphasis was on the use of bronchodilators prior to BPH and positioning. Breathing exercises focused on use of the supine and upright positions, facilitation of diaphragmatic control, maximum inspiratory hold, and progressive strength training of the inspiratory muscles. Bed mobility, bed to chair transfers, and low level ambulation were also included. All activity training incorporated breathing control activities. Medical treatment involved gentle diuresing, removal of the chest tube, platelet transfusion for a hematocrit below 30, continued antibiotic therapy, and placement of a gastrostomy tube to improve her nutritional status. The long-term goal was to wean the patient from ventilatory support. Methods used incorporated a team approach, combining a slow initial decrease in the rate of IMV as her strength gradually improved (demonstrated by an increase in inspiratory force). Progress included a gradual increase in the time the patient would breathe on her own with longer periods of sitting.

First Time Out of Intensive Care

By May 15 the patient was off all ventilatory support. She was transferred out of the ICU on June 11. At rest initially she was tachypneic, with a paradoxical breathing pattern. The tracheostomy tube remained in place because the team concluded she would not be able to manage the increased WOB as a result of the increase in upper airway dead space without it. She required minimal assistance of one for transfers and was walking short distances with a rolling walker.

Measurement of Outcome. Three days later on June 14 the patient began to complain of left-side numbness and weakness. This was accompanied by an increase in respiratory distress and increased sputum production. Her chest x-ray showed an elevated left hemidiaphragm but no new infiltrate. Her ABG values deteriorated to 81/81/7.20. A CT scan of her brain showed no new infarct. Possible causes for respiratory failure were mucus plugging, $\dot{V}_A:\dot{Q}$ mismatch, and hypercarbia. Later in the day an ABG on 60 percent O_2 via a trach mask was 122/91/7.17. The patient was manually hyperinflated with a 100 percent O_2 hand resuscitator and transferred back to the ICU for another long stay. During this time her blood pressure and kidney function remained within reasonable limits.

The patient once again underwent a slow weaning process. This time she was provided with nocturnal positive pressure ventilation to assist with diaphragmatic fatigue. By July 27 her RR was 20 to 32 on 50 percent O_2 via a tracheal mask and she was off all ventilatory support. On August 9 she was taken to the operating room and underwent a cholecystectomy and diaphragmatic plication. Once she recovered from the surgery she was transferred to a collaborative care nursing unit on September 3.

At this time she required contact guarding for all transfers and ambulation. She was able to walk 120 feet with a walker but required frequent rest periods. Her HR was in the 90s, with occasional premature atrial and ventricular contractions. She demonstrated problems with orthostatic hypotension. Her SBP was 140 mmHg supine, 108 mmHg sitting, and 98 mmHg standing. At rest her RR was 24, and her SaO_2 was 95 percent on room air. Approximately 4 weeks past the diaphragmatic plication her PFT values were FVC, 1.28 L (41 percent); FEV_1, .82 L (32 percent); and FEV_1:FVC ratio, 64 percent. Pulmonary mechanics were inspiratiory force, -60 mmHg; Vt, 250 ml; and VC, 1.1 L. Her chest x-ray still showed an elevated left hemidiaphragm. The tube feedings were meeting 90 percent of her caloric needs, although she was having frequent problems with diarrhea. Her renal function was beginning to deteriorate, with a BUN of 114 and a creatinine of 8.6

Reassessment.   Mobilizing secretions, decreasing the WOB, and maintaining functional mobility remained short-term goals. Her pulmonary hygiene was now being carried out by the nursing staff. Strengthening exercises and ambulation were also part of her daily routine.

Exercise Prescription

On September 12 the patient participated in a low level exercise test that was performed on a cycle ergometer. The purpose of the test was to determine if she were capable of training for cardiovascular endurance. The results of the test are shown in Table 9-5. The test was terminated at 2 minutes due to general fatigue. Oxygen was provided by 40 percent face mask throughout the test. Her BP and HR response were normal and she did not desaturate. Since her MVV was below her predicted voluntary ventilation of 28 L/min, she did not reach her ventilatory limit. Consequently, the therapist determined she could potentially benefit from an endurance exercise program. The short-term goal was now to increase her functional capacity.

The patient began a twice per day program of cycle ergometry using 2-minute intermittent cycling/rest segments for a total of 8 minutes cycling. Within a few weeks the patient was tolerating an interval training program

Table 9-5. Results of Exercise Test for Case Study #2

Stage	HR (beats per minute)	BP	RR	SaO$_2$ (%)	$\dot{V}e$	Comments
Resting	100	150/84	34	97	—	Test terminated due to general fatigue; secretions cleared throughout session.
1 minute of cycling	107	162/80	54	96	7.5	
2 minutes of cycling	110	160/80	60	99	10.8	

Abbreviations: HR, heart rate; BP, blood pressure; RR, respiratory rate; SaO$_2$, oxygen saturation; $\dot{V}e$, ventilation.

on the cycle ergometer to include 10 minutes of cycling alternating with 1 minute of rest for a total cycling time of 20 minutes. Vital signs were stable during exercise but she did exhibit a hypotensive response immediately postexercise that corrected itself within a few minutes of rest. Her RR went from 20 at rest to 45 with maximum exercise. Her HR went from 88 bpm at rest to 108 bpm at maximum exercise. She would also clear a large amount of secretions after each session. She began gradually tolerating a trach button for 10 minutes at a time and was walking longer distances with the nursing staff. The long-term goal was now to plan for discharge from the hospital by late November.

Measurement of Outcome. Although the patient and her family did manage a 1-day home visit in December, her chronic renal failure worsened and she became dependent upon dialysis. On December 11 an arteriovenostomy was performed for placement of a shunt. She continued to have problems with pulmonary sepsis but became unresponsive to antibiotic therapy. She also developed a gastrointestinal bleed due to a duodenal ulcer documented by endoscopy. During the last week in December she became unresponsive. The family decided that resuscitation measures were not to be administered should cardiac or pulmonary arrest occur. The patient died on January 1.

CASE STUDY #3

The patient is a 57-year-old man with a 66 pack-year smoking history. He began smoking cigarettes at age 12 and averaged 2 packs per day for 33 years. He quit smoking at age 55 because of shortness of breath with stair climbing. He developed pneumonia at age 14 and states he has had a daily productive cough since then. His occupational history is significant in that he was a firefighter for 15 years. At the age of 42 he again developed pneumonia. He was told then that according to his chest x-ray he had emphysema. He experienced a spontaneous pneumothorax at 56 years of age that was successfully treated with a chest tube. After that hospitalization he referred himself to a physician specializing in pulmonary medicine due to continued shortness of breath with minimal activity. The only other medical history is that of hypertension that had been temporarily treated 4 years earlier.

His PFT values, listed in Table 9-6, showed severe obstructive disease with moderate decrease in diffusion capacity. Room air ABG values were 62/40/7.42 (values:PaO_2, $PaCO_2$, pH). His chest x-ray demonstrated flattened diaphragms, bullous changes, enlarged proximal pulmonary arteries, narrowed peripheral vessels, and an enlarged heart. An exercise test was performed on a treadmill to evaluate the possibility of oxygen desaturation with activity. The patient was able to complete one stage of exercise at 2 mph and 0 percent grade. SaO_2 went from 89 percent at rest to 86 percent at the end of stage 1. The same workload was repeated with 2 L O_2. SaO_2 levels then remained above 92 percent. His $\dot{V}e$ was 52.1 L, which was greater than his predicted MVV. His physician recommended portable oxygen to be used with all daily activities. The patient refused, stating that having to use oxygen would be too depressing.

He was started on a program of broncholilator therapy to include Theo-Dur, 600 mg bid, and a Ventolin inhaler, 2 puffs qid. He was also referred to chest physical therapy for an outpatient pulmonary rehabilitation program.

Evaluation

Observation. The patient presented as obese, arriving for his first clinical visit in no respiratory distress. His breathing pattern was coordinated with diaphragmatic use at rest. Maximal inspiration resulted in the use of his upper chest and accessory muscles.

Patient Interview. Patient was a good historian and willing to communicate. He complained of shortness of breath with one flight of stairs or walking a half-mile on an average day. During periods of extreme temperature changes, hot or cold, his shortness of breath was worse. He stated he had a cough that was productive throughout the day, in addition to severe episodes that lasted for at least 10 minutes every night when he lay down to go to sleep. All these symptoms had increased significantly since his last hospitalization. He stated that on a daily basis he was trying to do as little walking as possible. He was living with a very supportive wife in a large 10-room home. He was the father of eight children, five of whom were still

Table 9-6. Pulmonary Function Test for Case Study #3

Test	Actual Measure	Percent of Predicted Measure
Forced vital capacity (FVC)	3.75 L	75
Forced expiratory volume for one second (FEV_1)	1.46 L	41
Ratio of FEV_1: FVC	39%	55
Residual volume (RV)	3.25 L	130
Total lung capacity (TLC)	7.14 L	95
Ratio of RV:TLC	46%	139
Diffusion capacity (DLCO)		59

living at home, the youngest being 19 years old. He was still employed by the fire department but had spent the past 20 years as a building inspector. At times this required his climbing three flights of stairs, which he stated was extremely difficult for him to do. He admitted to an alcohol intake of 8 to 12 cans of beer per day. He had cut back to 1 to 2 cans for the past 2 weeks in preparation for beginning the rehabilitation program.

Physical Examination. Vital signs at rest were a BP of 170/84, a HR of 90 bpm, a RR of 18, and an SaO_2 of 89 percent. Palpation revealed an inspiratory to expiratory ratio of 1:2, an increased anteroposterior to lateral diameter ratio of 1:1, a subcostal angle of 110 degrees, and no posterior excursion. Breath sounds were with poor aeration and coarse rales scattered throughout both lower lobes. He was 6 feet tall and weighed 268 pounds. He had two-pillow orthopnea and no swelling in his ankles.

Assessment and Goals

It was decided that certain clinical problems needed to be addressed prior to beginning an exercise program. Goals were set to improve airway patency, which in turn would have some effect on his hypoxemia and shortness of breath. It was also important to monitor his blood pressure over a period of time to determine if treatment of hypertension would be required prior to beginning an exercise program. The clinical problems, goals, and treatment plans are listed in Table 9-7.

Table 9-7. Clinical Problems and Treatment Plan for Case Study #3

Clinical Problems	Treatment Plan
Copious sputum production	Bronchodilator therapy
STG: decrease sputum production, improve airway patency	Postural drainage with breathing exercises
	Percussion and shaking
LTG: decrease hypoxemia, decrease shortness of breath	Home program with family assistance
	Position of relaxation
Consult physician	Antibiotic therapy if indicated
Shortness of breath with low level activity	Education: mechanics of breathing, position
STG: improve breathing pattern with activity	of relaxation, controlled breathing patterns,
LTG: decrease shortness of breath	proper use of broncholidator
Hypertension	Education: risk factors
STG: decrease alcohol intake	Emotional support
LTG: lose weight, decrease blood pressure	Referral to nutritionist if indicated
Obesity	
STG: lose weight	Education: changes in daily dietary and
LTG: decrease blood pressure	alcoholic intake.
	Emotional support
	Referral to nutritionist
Deconditioning	
STG: 20 consecutive minutes of exercise	Education: need for long-term compliance
LTG: 30 consecutive minutes of exercise with target HR of 115–137 bpm, begin independent home program	Endurance exercise program on stationary bicycle

Abbreviations: STG, short-term goals; LTG, long-term goals; HR, heart rate; bpm, beats per minute.

Treatment, Measurement of Outcome, and Reassessment

The patient was seen in the outpatient clinic 3 times per week for BPH, which included bronchodilator therapy, postural drainage, and manual techniques. During the first week he was also instructed in controlled breathing patterns with walking and stair climbing, as well as in a home program of postural drainage and breathing exercises. To enhance the home program his wife was taught manual techniques during the second week of treatment.

Measurement of Outcome.   With each clinic visit a copious amount of green sputum was produced and breath sounds improved with increased aeration but persistent rales. The patient and his wife were noncompliant with the home program. After 2 weeks there was no significant change in the color or amount of sputum he was producing.

Reassessment.   His physician was consulted and the patient was started on a 2-week course of antibiotics (Ampicillin).

Measurement of Outcome.   The program of BPH continued throughout the antibiotic therapy. Significant improvement was noted during that time. Much less sputum was produced and it changed to pale yellow. The patient stated that he continued to have episodes of productive coughing at night but that he presently was doing very little coughing during the day. His breath sounds were consistent with improved aeration throughout and his SaO_2 had increased to 93 percent at rest. His PFT results were unchanged. He had minimized his alcohol intake to a few beers on weekends and his BP had decreased to 150/74. It was now felt that the patient was ready to begin an exercise program. The results of the exercise test are shown in Table 9-8.

Assessment and Goals

The exercise test was performed on a stationary bicycle in 6-minute stages. The patient was able to complete 4 minutes of stage 2 at a workload of 75 W. The test was terminated because the patient felt he could not breathe and his legs were extremely fatigued. He reached his exercise limitation at a very low maximum HR of 116 bpm. His BP response to exercise was hypertensive, with a maximum BP of 232/112. His ECG remained in normal sinus rhythm, with occasional premature ventricular contractions during stage 2. His $\dot{V}e$ was 56.3 L, which exceeded his predicted MVV. His SaO_2 remained above 90 percent. The interpretation of the exercise test was that he exhibited both a pulmonary and cardiovascular limitation to exercise. The major benefit of an exercise program would be the reversal of his extreme deconditioning.

Treatment, Measurement of Outcome, and Reassessment

The patient was started on a supervised exercise program. Each session included a treatment of BPH prior to exercise on a stationary bicycle.

Table 9-8. Results of Exercise Test for Case Study #3

Stage	Time (minutes)	HR (beats per minute)[a]	BP	RR	SaO_2 (%)	Comments
Resting		89	156/66	20	93	
Stage 1						
.5 KP	2	102	190/92	30	93	
50 rpm	4	102	202/98	30	93	At the end of stage 1, he complained of some leg fatigue but
25 W	6	103	180/100	30	92	felt he could continue to exercise.
	1 $\overline{p}$	93	150/90	24	94	
	5 $\overline{p}$	89	150/84	24	94	
Stage 2						
1.5 KP	2	110	184/110	30	90	Stage 2 terminated after 4 minutes due to shortness of breath
50 rpm	4	116	232/112	30	90	and leg fatigue. Breathing pattern remained coordinated
75 W	1 $\overline{p}$	101	200/98	24	93	with significant increase in work of breathing noted.
	5 $\overline{p}$	97	160/90	24	93	
Posttest	2 $\overline{p}$	102	130/80	12	96	

Abbreviations: HR, heart rate; BP, blood pressure; RR, respiratory rate; SaO_2, oxygen saturation; KP, kiloponds; rpm, revolutions per minute; W, watts; $\overline{p}$, posttest.

[a] Predicted maximum heart rate was 163 beats per minute.

Although he continued to do very little coughing throughout his daily activities his cough was consistently productive during the treatments and after each exercise session. He remained noncompliant with a home program for secretion clearance. At the beginning of the exercise program his weight was still 266 pounds. His alcohol intake was much less and BP at rest equaled 140/74. The patient refused to meet with a nutritionist. He stated that he and his wife were aware of what needed to be done; they merely had to make a commitment to the necessary changes.

Week One

His initial exercise prescription was as follows: an intensity of 37.5 W, a duration of 13 consecutive minutes, and a frequency of 3 times per week.

Measurement of Outcome. His most limiting factor to the above exercise was leg fatigue. His HR ranged between 109 and 112 bpm, maximum BP was 186/100, maximum RR was 30, and SaO_2 remained above 89 percent. Occasional premature ventricular contractions were noted.

Reassessment. A preferred target HR for this patient during exercise would have been 114 to 137 bpm (70 to 85 percent of predicted maximum HR); however, he was not able to reach that intensity level. Emphasis was initially placed on the duration of the exercise prescription in order to reach the short-term goal of 20 consecutive minutes of cycling. This was accomplished by having the patient exercise at an HR less than 70 percent of a predicted maximum. By the end of the first week he was able to exercise for 15 consecutive minutes, with a maximum HR of 113 bpm.

Week Three

Measurement of Outcome. He no longer complained of leg fatigue at the end of each session but he did feel short of breath and tired. His HR ranged between 114 and 119 bpm, maximum BP was 200/90, and maximum RR was 30.

Reassessment. The exercise prescription was advanced as follows: an intensity of 50 W, duration of 20 consecutive minutes, and a frequency of 3 times per week. It was felt the patient was progressing well.

Week Five

Measurement of Outcome. His cough remained productive of pale yellow secretions primarily after exercise and at night when he went to bed. His wife was willing to assist with a home program of BPH but the patient remained unwilling to carry this out. It appeared that he did not want to put himself in a dependent role. The exercise prescription was tolerated with a maximum HR of 115 bpm, maximum BP of 196/90, maximum RR of 30, and an SaO_2 above 88 percent. His weight was 264 pounds and his resting BP was 150/60. He subjectively began to notice less shortness of breath with ambulation.

Reassessment. The exercise prescription remained unchanged. The patient continued to perceive this workload as difficult. A stationary bicycle had been purchased for home use and both the therapist and the patient felt he would be able to continue the exercise program independently at home for 1 month.

Return Visit

The patient had maintained a commitment to the exercise program and was riding his stationary bicycle 3 times per week for 25 minutes. He was also walking a half-mile 1 to 2 times per week. His cough and sputum production remained unchanged. He had resumed his daily alcohol intake and 1 week previous to this clinic visit his BP had been 170/84. This issue was addressed at pulmonary rehabilitation rounds as a significant factor for limiting progress. His physician agreed and addressed the alcohol issue very directly. The patient has now not had any alcohol for the past week.

Measurement of Outcome. After a month of an independent home program his vital signs at rest were BP, 130/84; HR, 71 bpm; RR, 18; and SaO_2, 91 percent. His weight remained 266 pounds. The workload of 50 W resulted in a maximum HR of 101 bpm and a maximum BP of 180/84.

Reassessment. He was instructed to increase the workload on the stationary bicycle to 62.5 W and we reviewed the proper technique for monitoring his own heart rate. Once again emphasis was placed on his need to commit himself to all other aspects of the program, such as losing weight and not drinking alcohol. The patient once again refused assistance in dealing with these issues. It was felt by both the therapist and the patient that in order to maintain and improve his compliance with the program he should return in 3 months for another reevaluation.

Discharge

When the patient returned in 3 months, the major improvement was that he had lost 32 pounds. He had minimal complaint of shortness of breath throughout his daily activities. His cough remained productive only after exercise and at night. He was riding his stationary bicycle 3 times per week for 25 minutes at the same workload. At rest his vital signs were BP, 140/76; HR, 87 bpm; RR, 18; and SaO_2, 92 percent. With exercise they were maximum BP, 180/86; maximum HR, 115 bpm; maximum RR, 26; his SaO_2 remained above 90 percent. He admitted to continued alcohol intake of one six-pack of beer per day and more on weekends.

Since the beginning of the program he had doubled his exercise tolerance from 32 W for 13 minutes to 62 W for 25 minutes. His complaints of shortness of breath and cough with sputum production were minimal. His BP was within a good range and he had lost some weight. It was felt that most of the goals from Table 9-7 had been reached and he was discharged to continue with his home program independently.

REFERENCES

1. Ramsden EL: Bases for clinical decision making: perception of the patient, the clinician's role and responsibility. p. 21. In Wolf SL (ed): Clinical Decision Making in Physical Therapy. FA Davis, Philadelphia, 1985
2. Magistro CM: Clinical decision making in physical therapy: a practitioner's perspective. Phys Ther 69:525, 1989
3. Hislop HJ: Clinical decision making: educational, data and risk factors. p. 25. Wolf SL (ed): Clinical Decision Making in Physical Therapy. FA Davis, Philadelphia, 1985
4. Watts NT: Decision analysis: a tool for improving physical therapy practice and education. p. 7. Wolf SL (ed): Clinical Decision Making in Physical Therapy. FA Davis, Philadelphia, 1985
5. Holden MK: Clinical decision making among neurologic patients: stroke. p. 171. Wolf SL (ed): Clinical Decision Making in Physical Therapy. FA Davis, Philadelphia, 1985
6. Johnson GR: Bases for clinical decision making: assimilating data and marketing skills. p. 61. Wolf SL (ed): Clinical Decision Making in Physical Therapy. FA Davis, Philadelphia, 1985

Index

Page numbers followed by f *indicate figures; those followed by* t *indicate tables.*